PRAISE FOR
THE ROAD TO ... CULTURES

"This elegant and charming book focuses on the realities of today's nursing workplace culture. Drawn from Dr. Huston's experience as an authentic leader in a variety of work settings and synthesized into 10 easy-to-learn leadership lessons, the book gives readers insight into their own workplace culture and offers practical strategies to improve it. Traveling this road with her as a guide is a must for students, emerging leaders, and any nurse who is currently in a leadership position."

–Diane M. Billings, EdD, RN, ANEF, FAAN
Chancellor's Professor Emeritus
Indiana University School of Nursing, Indianapolis

"Dr. Huston's new book presents a tremendous resource of relevant and practical guidance for transforming work culture. Her book is valuable because it is amazingly timely, given the challenges nurse leaders face in today's social climate, and because it presents well-proven truths and approaches that are of lasting value and applicable in many environments. She has thoughtfully selected clear and compelling material that will become an essential resource for any nurse leader who aspires to be an agent of positive change."

–Sheila Burke, DNP, MBA, MSN, NEA-BC
Vice President, Nursing Education Affiliates Inc.

THE ROAD TO
POSITIVE
WORK
CULTURES

CAROL J. HUSTON, DPA, MSN, RN, FAAN

To order additional books, buy in bulk, or order for corporate use, contact Sigma Marketplace at 888.654.4968 (US and Canada) or +1.317.634.8171 (outside US and Canada).

To request a review copy for course adoption, email solutions@sigmamarketplace.org or call 888.654.4968 (US and Canada) or +1.317.634.8171 (outside US and Canada).

To request author information, or for speaker or other media requests, contact Sigma Marketing at 888.634.7575 (US and Canada) or +1.317.634.8171 (outside US and Canada).

ISBN: 9781948057417
EPUB ISBN: 9781948057424
PDF ISBN: 9781948057431
MOBI ISBN: 9781948057448

Library of Congress Control Number: 2019947826

First Printing, 2019

Publisher: Dustin Sullivan

Acquisitions Editor: Emily Hatch

Series Cover Design: Rebecca Batchelor

Cover Designer: TnT Design

Interior Design/Page Layout: Rebecca Batchelor

Managing Editor: Carla Hall

Publications Specialist: Todd Lothery

Copy Editor: Jane Palmer

Proofreader: Todd Lothery

Indexer: Jane Palmer

ACKNOWLEDGMENTS

I would like to acknowledge and thank the many mentors, role models, colleagues, family members, and friends who have shaped my personal leadership journey. Your support, guidance, and love have made such a difference.

ABOUT THE AUTHOR

Carol J. Huston, DPA, MSN, RN, FAAN

Carol J. Huston has been a professor in the School of Nursing at California State University, Chico (CSUC) since 1982 and assumed the position of Director of the School of Nursing from 2010–15. She currently teaches classes on leadership, management, health finance, and health systems part time as emerita professor. Huston was named one of seven CSUC Master Teachers in 1999, 2000, and 2001; the CSUC Outstanding Teacher for the 2001–02 academic year; and the CSUC Outstanding Professor for the 2008–09 academic year.

Huston is author or coauthor of seven textbooks on leadership, management, and professional issues in nursing (a total of 22 editions) as well as a children's book, *When Little Girls Dream*. She is author of *The Road to Leadership*, published by Sigma Theta Tau International Honor Society of Nursing (Sigma) in 2017. The fifth edition of *Professional Issues in Nursing: Challenges and Opportunities* published in 2019. Her coauthored book *Leadership Roles and Management Functions in Nursing* has been translated into four languages and received a 2017 AJN Book of the Year award. The 10th edition of that book will publish in 2020. Huston has also published more than 100 articles and editorials in leading professional journals.

In addition, Huston has given more than 300 presentations at nursing and healthcare conferences worldwide. She is also a successful grant writer and has been the primary investigator or coinvestigator of multiple grants. Huston has served on the Enloe Medical Center (Chico, California) board of trustees since 2012 and as Chair of the board since 2016.

Huston is a Fellow in the American Academy of Nursing. In addition, she served as the 2007–09 President of Sigma. As President, she was responsible for strategic planning, program implementation, and fiduciary oversight of approximately 130,000 nurses in more than 470 chapters located in more than 90 countries. Huston also served as Co-chair of the 2010 International Year of the Nurse (IYNurse) Initiative, a global partnership effort of Sigma, the Nightingale Initiative for Global Health, and the Nightingale Museum of London. She served as lead faculty for Sigma's Experienced Nurse Faculty Leadership Academy from 2014 to 2019 and is a consultant for Sigma's Institute for Global Healthcare Leadership, which launched in Washington, DC, in September 2016.

TABLE OF CONTENTS

PREFACE

This book was written to foster the development of leadership skills that create and sustain positive work cultures. Cultures are the shared values and beliefs that guide thinking and behavior (Eades, 2018). Current evidence suggests that many nurses work in cultures that at best are not supportive and at worst, toxic. Indeed, the expectation that nurses will receive the same care and kindness in the workplace that they give to their patients is often not the case.

That's because positive work cultures don't happen by accident. They exist because of the hard work of many people, but especially individuals who hold both formal and informal leadership roles in that culture. The fact is, leaders must constantly work to shape positive work cultures because they are often responsible for them.

This book, then, is about strategies leaders can use to actively create and then sustain positive work cultures. It describes what a positive workplace culture looks like, why it is needed, and how to achieve it. Emphasis is placed on the leader's role in making that happen as well as the challenges that arise when values are in conflict or when individual needs and wants supersede those of the team.

"**Culture is everything to a team, and while everyone on the team plays a part in the ongoing development of the culture, it's the leader's responsibility to create and mold it.**"

—John Eades

Many of the chapters include personal insights gained from my own leadership experiences, and I have purposefully shared situations where other people or I encountered frustration or failure as a leader. My hope in sharing these stories is that readers will recognize that leadership is a journey and not a destination—and that although missteps occur, leaders who are authentic and create atmospheres of mutual respect, trust, and appreciation can positively impact the work cultures of others.

Chapter 1 begins with a discussion about characteristics of positive work cultures, why leaders matter in creating positive work cultures, and the challenges of creating a shared vision and goals when subcultures are present.

Chapter 2 focuses on the importance of establishing a climate of mutual respect and civility, suggesting that the responsibility for dealing with incivility lies with both frontline staff and the organization because zero tolerance must be the expectation.

Chapter 3 examines why leaders must establish boundaries to separate their responsibility from what belongs to others—and to eliminate as much confusion as possible about their role as "boss" versus that of friend or colleague. This chapter also presents boundaries as a space that allows leaders to separate their beliefs and actions from others—because the leader cannot always control how others feel or behave.

Chapter 4 suggests that avoiding micromanagement is critical to the establishment and maintenance of positive work cultures. Instead of micromanaging, leaders should macromanage and empower workers to be innovative and creative in identifying new ways to solve problems or complete delegated tasks.

Chapter 5 observes that in positive work cultures, managers address organizational problems as soon as they occur. Often, these problems are related to interpersonal or team conflict, but they may include the need for employee disciplinary action or behavior modification.

Chapter 6 examines the importance of effective teams in building positive work cultures. Building trust by establishing genuine relationships with workers, exhibiting integrity, being transparent, and demonstrating competence also further team-building efforts. In addition, leaders must be effective communicators and role-model excellent communication skills for teams to flourish.

Chapter 7 focuses on the importance of leaders addressing and reducing workload stress for employees whenever possible. Dynamic change is a significant part of most contemporary organizational cultures. Thus, leaders must first assure that change is happening for a good reason and then help workers understand how changes will impact their lives. Leaders must also support employees during these changes and give them as much control as possible over working conditions. Finally, leaders must always assure that the workload is reasonable.

Chapter 8 suggests that showing appreciation and rewarding desired behavior are critical in building positive work cultures. Often, this is as simple as leaders recognizing workers for a job well done, but it also may include providing other types of incentives or rewards that have value to those they are leading.

Chapter 9 addresses the importance of authentic leadership in creating positive work cultures. This requires leaders to be transparent, to demonstrate consistency between stated values and actions, and to be self-aware about the values that are driving their actions.

Finally, **Chapter 10** speaks to the importance of vision, passion, and purpose as tools leaders can use to promote positive work cultures. When leaders continually look to the future, embrace change, create an action plan to achieve their vision, and inspire followers with passion, organizations become ever-renewing.

"We are what we
repeatedly do.
Excellence, then,
is not an act,
but a habit."

—Will Durant

"You manage things; you lead people."

—Rear Admiral Grace Hopper

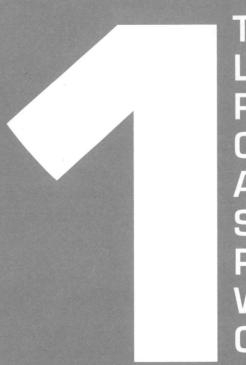

1

THE
LEADER'S
ROLE IN
CREATING
AND
SUSTAINING
POSITIVE
WORK
CULTURES

One of the biggest challenges faced by organizations today is developing a collaborative and productive workplace culture that can boost performance. Indeed, *culture* is an important and complex part of every organization, representing an organization's values, belief systems, language, traditions, and customs. Culture provides the "feel" of an organization and determines what is right or wrong, important or unimportant, and workable or unworkable. In other words, culture is everywhere and affects everything. These beliefs and values, however, are rarely written down.

Kohll (2018) agrees, suggesting that culture affects nearly every aspect of an organization. From recruiting top talent to improving employee satisfaction, it's the backbone of a happy workforce. Without a positive organizational culture, many employees struggle to find the real value in their work, and this can lead to a variety of negative consequences.

Organizational culture is not the same, however, as *organizational climate*—how employees perceive an organization. For example, an employee might perceive an organization as fair, friendly, and informal or as formal and very structured. The perception may be accurate or inaccurate, and people in the same organization may have different perceptions about their organization. Therefore, because the organizational climate is from the viewpoint of individuals, the organization's climate and culture may differ.

And then, to complicate things further, larger organizations also have different and competing value systems that create *subcultures*. These subcultures shape their members' perceptions and attitudes toward work and the organization. For example, when I worked rotating shifts, I found that nurses from different shifts often complained about each other and about the work they perceived should have been accomplished and was not. This created a sense of "us versus them" and divided, rather than united, us as workers.

I have also experienced this with the assimilation of faculty. Some younger faculty are frustrated with curriculum change they perceive to be too slow, and some older faculty think young faculty are impatient and disrespectful. It's a delicate balance to recognize the wisdom and experience of the organization's most senior workers and, at the same time, seek the innovation and willingness to embrace change commonly seen in younger members of the workforce. A critical challenge, then, is for leaders to recognize these subcultures and do what is necessary to create a culture of shared norms and priorities.

Agarwal (2018) agrees, noting the importance of having clear organizational core values that are communicated effectively and shared by employees. A core value is the commitment that an organization or a company makes to certain policies and actions, such as "just cultures" or "promoting diversity." Agarwal says it is not enough to just state these values in the mission statement, brand story, or marketing and promotional material. Instead, organizations must regularly act on these values so that employees feel an individual and personal responsibility to do the same.

> **"Culture is about performance, and making people feel good about how they contribute to the whole."**
>
> —Tracy Streckenbach

For example, I once worked for a boss who talked all the time about the importance of leadership succession and development. But whenever an opportunity came up to delegate new or important tasks to employees to learn and grow from, he clung to those tasks. As a result, employees became demoralized because they felt he did not trust them to do the job right. Therefore, positive attitudes and positive actions make for a positive work culture, and the inverse is true as well.

How are cultures created in the first place? Certainly, individuals bring their values and belief systems to their workplaces. However, leadership and strategic organizational directions likely have the greatest impact. Founders and influential leaders often set new cultures in motion and imprint values and assumptions that persist for decades (Groysberg, Lee, Price, & Yo-Jud Cheng, 2018). Thus, leaders not only are instrumental in setting a tone for workplace culture but also do their work in a larger context and are influenced by existing culture in turn (Gartenstein, 2019, para 1).

> "Growing a culture requires a good storyteller. Changing a culture requires a persuasive editor."
>
> —Ryan Lilly

For example, Apple founders Steve Jobs and Steve Wozniak created a corporate philosophy that emphasized creative innovation, recognizable products, and simple design, and their organizational culture emphasized hiring only the best of the best in the labor market (Meyer, 2019). In addition, excellence was emphasized as a critical success factor—especially in product design and development, which was a major growth strategy. When Tim Cook took over as chief executive officer of Apple in 2011, he worked hard to maintain this culture and most of the values of his predecessor.

Over time, though, an organization's leaders can also shape culture through both conscious and unconscious actions—sometimes with unintended consequences. For example, the culture Jobs created at Apple also included moderate leadership combativeness (Meyer, 2019). However, Cook has been working to change this corporate culture to be more sociable and less combative.

The best leaders, then, "are fully aware of the multiple cultures within which they are embedded, can sense when change is required, and can deftly influence the process" (Groysberg et al., 2018, para. 3). Sustaining positive cultures is another goal. Thus, culture and leadership are inextricably linked.

What makes a work culture positive? Many things. For example, positive work cultures provide a high level of *employee engagement*, the term used to describe an employee's emotional commitment to the organization and its goals. When employees are highly engaged, they enjoy their work, find it meaningful, and work hard to achieve shared goals. They are also excited about the future because they know where they are headed and feel they can play a role in reaching important organizational goals. Feeling valued, being treated fairly, receiving feedback and direction, and having a strong working relationship between employee and manager that is based on mutual respect all contribute to employee engagement (Custom Insight, n.d.).

In addition, mutual respect, trust, and civility are core values in positive work cultures. Employees feel appreciated and empowered to solve problems at the level they occur. Opportunities exist for mentorship, personal and professional development, and career advancement. In addition, a team atmosphere is created when employees can work with organization leaders to set goals, make decisions, and implement change.

Open and honest communication also flows freely throughout positive work cultures, and divergence in thinking to improve organizational workflow is both encouraged and supported. Organizations with positive work cultures demonstrate that they value their employees, such as by providing flexible work schedules that fit employees' lives.

"Too many smart and capable people end up leaving their jobs not because of the work itself or the compensation plan, but because they were tired of pushing a rock uphill every working day."

—Liz Ryan

In contrast, a toxic or negative work culture exemplifies unhappiness, low motivation, and apathy. No one feels responsible. Instead, "the politics, the stupid rules and the dark, fearful energy" (Ryan, 2016, para. 2) flow throughout the workplace and bog everyone down so that little gets accomplished. Ryan notes that most people will only push so hard for so long before they stop and ask: "Why am I killing myself for this job? No one appreciates what I am doing. What am I trying to prove?" (para. 5). If there are no signs that things will get better anytime soon, they simply stop trying.

Although anyone can begin a conversation about the elephant in the room— a broken culture—almost everybody has an excuse for why they are not doing anything about it (Ryan, 2016). Some fear getting fired, others feel powerless to change a longstanding culture, and still others simply no longer have the energy to tackle what they see as a hopeless situation.

Building and sustaining a positive culture, particularly if a negative culture is in place, requires the interpersonal, team-building, and communication skills of a leader. The more entrenched the culture and pattern of actions, the more challenging the change process for the leader. This is where leadership really matters. Courage is a critical leadership skill, and risk-taking is a big part of courage. Negative or toxic work cultures will not change on their own; transforming such cultures requires the skills of a dedicated and courageous change champion.

When new leaders come into existing cultures, they have three choices: attempt to destroy it, nurture it, or evolve it (Solomon, 2018). The most appropriate response depends on the situation. Destroying the existing culture (and replacing it with something new) is both the most ambitious and the riskiest. But destruction and rebirth may be so important that failure to destroy the current culture will mean the ultimate death of the organization.

Surrendering to the existing culture is easier, although the ability to successfully steward and sustain that culture depends on its strength and viability. If the existing culture is strong, stewardship is easy. If it is weak, it becomes much harder.

Evolving the culture is frequently the best choice for leaders who want to effectively make changes (Solomon, 2018). In evolving the culture, what is good is embraced, and what is bad is replaced. It is not easy, however, because leadership and culture work bidirectionally (Solomon, 2018). Leadership can affect culture, and culture can overwhelm attempts at leadership, particularly when leaders attempt strategic changes. What ends up happening regarding culture depends on the strength of the leader, the strength of the culture, and the ambition of the leader's approach. Leaders who think they can impose their will on a culture often find out that the culture has other ideas.

"Culture eats strategy for breakfast."

—Peter Drucker

Bradberry (2017) suggests it may be helpful to remember that the first step in leading change is always the hardest. Once you take that step, anxiety and fear often dissipate in the name of action. "People that dive headfirst into taking that brutal first step aren't any stronger than the rest of us; they've simply learned that it yields great results … and that procrastination only prolongs their suffering" (para. 7). No one wants to work in an organization with a negative culture; isn't it better to take on the risk to make things better than to sit back and accept a situation where you could have made a difference?

"When facing obstacles, you must decide if you're going to let them be the excuse for your failure or if you're going to make them the story behind your success."

–Travis Bradberry

"Employees engage with employers and brands when they're treated as humans worthy of respect."

—Meghan M. Biro

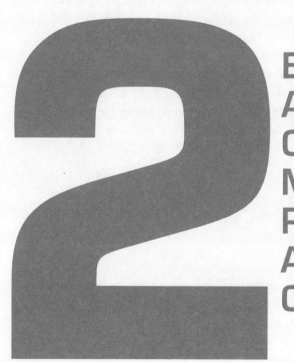

2

ESTABLISH
A CULTURE
OF
MUTUAL
RESPECT
AND
CIVILITY

The first strategy leaders can use to create and sustain positive work cultures is to establish a climate of mutual respect and civility. Indeed, the Society for Human Resource Management (2017) found that, "For the third year in a row, the largest percentage of respondents have indicated that respectful treatment of all employees at all levels was a very important contributor to their job satisfaction." Similarly, a recent survey of nearly 20,000 employees worldwide by Georgetown University's Christine Porath (as cited in Rogers, 2018) found that what mattered to them most was feeling respected by superiors. In fact, respondents ranked respect as the most important leadership behavior.

Heathfield (2018) defines *respect* as feelings of admiration and deep regard for an individual. You believe that the person has good qualities and capabilities and is worthy of your regard and admiration. When you respect individuals, then, you value them and recognize that they have rights, opinions, wishes, experience, and competence.

For example, I currently serve on the board of trustees for our local medical center. I truly respect the CEO because he displays so many of the values I want to emulate: openness, honesty, integrity, willingness to consider different points of view, and genuine interest in and caring about the staff and patients. He also respects and appreciates board members, encouraging them to "chafe" the senior leadership team with critical questions when they think there might be a different way to look at things, or if they believe a different course of action might be indicated.

What, then, does a climate of *mutual respect* look like? Besner (2015) says it means treating others as though they really matter. Brown (2018) says mutual respect is demonstrated by speaking to one another in a respectful and considerate fashion, keeping others in mind when making decisions, and responding to the needs and wants of others. It also means communicating respectfully, openly, and honestly, even when this is difficult. It does not mean consensus, as some divergence in thinking is critical for growth and innovation.

Not everyone feels secure enough, however, to embrace divergent thinking. A member of a social club board I serve on recently accused other board members of being disrespectful when they disagreed with how he felt about a board decision. It wasn't a case of disrespect, however. Board members encouraged him to voice his minority opinion, listened carefully, and acknowledged his opinion—but in the end, the board decided to vote differently. Indeed, I would argue that the dissenting board member was being disrespectful by not recognizing the right of others to have an opinion different from his own.

Organizational cultures can run the gamut, ranging from being disrespectful to highly respectful. This measure is not, however, static over time. Leaders can create organizational cultures where mutual respect becomes a core value—one that is understood, articulated, internalized, and acted upon by employees at all levels of the organization.

"Aspire to decency. Practice civility toward one another. Admire and emulate ethical behavior wherever you find it. Apply a rigid standard of morality to your lives; and if, periodically, you fail—as you surely will—adjust your lives, not the standards."

–Ted Koppel

What does a climate of *civility* look like? In its simplest, modern form, civility refers to politeness or showing regard for others. However, Tomas Spath and Cassandra Dahnke (n.d.), founders of the Institute for Civility in Government, suggest that civility is "claiming and caring for one's identity, needs and beliefs without degrading someone else's in the process" (para. 1). Thus, civility is not passive. A climate of civility does not mean that everyone agrees on everything. It means that people can address their differences assertively and respectfully and that everyone can be heard.

Likewise, *incivility* is the term used to describe mistreatment or discourtesy to another person. Clark (2017) sees incivility as a continuum—with disruptive behaviors, such as eye-rolling and other nonverbal behaviors and sarcastic comments, on one end and threatening behaviors, such as intimidation and physical violence, on the opposite end.

I have worked in cultures where employees were, at best, rude to each other. At worst, they were threatening to each other. This culture existed because it was the behavior role-modeled by our boss, who belittled employees, criticized them in front of others, and spoke incessantly about how much she hated her job and the "dregs" of human beings she had to manage. As a result, employees sabotaged her in both small and significant ways, and the culture became one of rampant disrespect.

Unfortunately, *bullying* is a frequent manifestation of incivility. The Workplace Bullying Institute (2019) defines bullying as repeated, health-harming mistreatment of one or more persons (the targets) by one or more perpetrators. The American Nurses Association (ANA) defines bullying as "repeated, unwanted, harmful actions intended to humiliate, offend, and cause distress in the recipient" (ANA, n.d., para. 2). Both definitions characterize bullying as abusive conduct that is threatening, humiliating, or intimidating in nature.

In addition, workplace incivility can be manifested by *mobbing*, when employees "gang up" on someone. The degree of harm a person experiences from bullying or mobbing depends on the frequency, intensity, and duration of the behavior or tactic used (Hockley, 2020). Moreover, what one person considers a harmful experience, another may not. Therefore, a person's experience with or perceptions about incivility are unique to that person.

Bullying, incivility, and mobbing that occur in the workplace are known as *workplace violence*. Verbal abuse is a common form of workplace violence against nurses. Hockley (2020) maintains, however, that workplace violence can also include physical violence—as well as various antisocial behaviors and incidents that lead people to believe that they have been harmed by the experience. These include, but are not limited to, behaviors such as engaging in favoritism, being verbally abusive, sending abusive correspondence, bullying, playing pranks, and setting workers up for failure. Workplace violence also includes economic aggression, such as denying opportunities for workers to be promoted.

Unfortunately, incivility is common in nursing. A 2017 ANA study of 10,688 RNs and student nurses found that about half of respondents had been bullied in some manner in the workplace, 25% had been physically assaulted at work by a patient or family member, and 9% were concerned for their physical safety at work. Unfortunately, as bad as these numbers are, they are likely much higher than reported. In fact, one survey estimated that just 19% of all workplace violence is reported (Douglas & Walasik, 2018).

While most nurses recognize the personal, emotional, and physical harm that often results from incivility, many don't realize that it also negatively impacts patient care. When any kind of violence is directed at nurses, they find it more difficult to remain committed to patient-centered care and to maintain ethical boundaries (Mann, 2018). These physical and psychological insults ultimately result in healthcare worker distraction, which contributes to a higher incidence of medication errors and negative patient outcomes (Locke, Bromley, & Federspiel, 2018). Other damaging consequences include moral distress, burnout, and job dissatisfaction, which can lead to increased turnover.

> **"Strong people stand up for themselves. Stronger people stand up for others."**
> —Chris Gardner

It's also true that far too often in nursing, we accept that some degree of incivility is just part of the job. For example, I've personally observed hand-off sessions that were more about bashing coworkers than they were about the patients. And I think at least some of us graduated from nursing schools at a time when physician behavior was above reproach, no matter how awful it really was, and when our female socialization kept us from responding in the assertive manner that we should have.

For example, early in my career, I saw a physician strike a nurse across the back with a metal chart when he became frustrated with her. The worst part was that while many of us saw it, none of us did anything. It was battery, and while the physician was verbally reprimanded, nothing further happened.

The responsibility for dealing with incivility should initially lie with frontline staff, but organizational leaders must become involved if the problem is not immediately resolved. In addition, organizations should have an anti-bullying policy in place that clearly describes zero tolerance as the expectation because bullying and incivility impact turnover, productivity, and quality of care. The policy should clearly define what behaviors and actions the organization considers inappropriate and what the consequences will be if the policy is violated.

"Zero tolerance should be the expectation because bullying and incivility impact turnover, productivity, and quality of care."

—Bessie Marquis & Carol Huston

In addition, all healthcare organizations have a responsibility to establish strategies for preventing workplace violence. Providing education, offering safety tips, maintaining a safe workplace environment, creating a plan of action, educating the public, and urging nurses to report perpetrators demonstrate that interventions reduce the occurrence of violence toward nurses (Mann, 2018). Employees are responsible for being open and willing to learn and implementing these interventions in their everyday practices.

Leaders must protect those who cannot protect themselves. Bullies must be immediately confronted, no matter how scary that may be, because incivility has no place in a professional work environment. And there must be consequences for individuals if the bullying behavior continues—because even one person can negatively impact the attitude of an entire work unit.

Bullying and incivility are never OK. It is up to each person to find the moral courage to recognize, report, and stop bullying and incivility. When you do not, you're condoning unprofessional behavior. Positive work cultures can exist only when leaders recognize that incivility should never occur and communicate that message to employees.

"The American Nurses Association (ANA) position statement on incivility, bullying, and workplace violence states that 'all registered nurses and employers in all settings, including practice, academia, and research must collaborate to create a culture of respect, free of incivility, bullying, and workplace violence.' In other words, violence should never be an accepted part of practice."

—Julia Mason Jubb & Cathryn J. Baack

"Boundaries are a part of self-care. They are healthy, normal, and necessary."

—Doreen Virtue

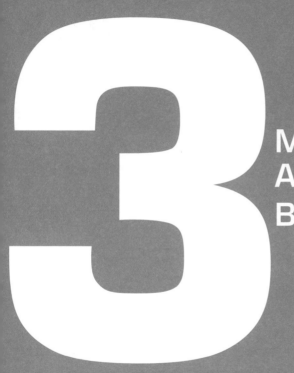

3
MAINTAIN APPROPRIATE BOUNDARIES

Another strategy that leaders can use to create a positive work culture is to maintain appropriate *boundaries*. Boundaries are the limits we set to protect ourselves. They can be fairly rigid or loose. Martin (2018b) suggests that boundaries are imaginary lines that separate your physical space, feelings, needs, and responsibilities from others. Your boundaries also tell other people how they can treat you—what's acceptable and what isn't. Without boundaries, people may take advantage of you because you haven't set limits on how you expect to be treated.

For example, I have created a boundary on social media between my personal and professional relationships. While I accept connections on my LinkedIn account from almost all healthcare-related, interdisciplinary colleagues, I limit my Facebook connections to close friends and family. This differentiates what I post on each site and what information each group can access.

Implementing boundaries, however, can sometimes be confusing to others. It might be helpful to remember that boundaries are intended to foster a healthy connection, not lead to relational disconnect or cutoff. "Boundaries communicate safety—and figuratively demarcate where I end, and you begin. Thus, boundaries allow us to make clear what is our responsibility and what is not. Much emotional turmoil and distress comes from taking on what is not ours, or letting others take responsibility for what is actually ours" (Chun, 2018, para. 10).

Another boundary is physical. All of us have some degree of personal distance that we consider to be a "safe space" between ourselves and others. This distance can vary by individual, though, particularly in relation to cultural differences. For example, I remember a former student who frequently attempted to put his arm around or touch his peers and, sometimes, even the faculty. He did not pick up the subtle clues most people are attuned to—that his behavior was making them feel uncomfortable. In fact, direct and repeated confrontation was required for his behavior to stop. Similarly, I am a "hugger," and I must be vigilant that my desire or propensity to hug someone to provide support or encouragement might be crossing their personal space boundary or be misinterpreted in some way.

Indeed, boundaries are essential to healthy relationships—and, really, a healthy life. Setting and sustaining boundaries are skills, however, that many people don't have. With people who have similar communication styles, views, personalities, and general approach to life, it may be easy (Tartakovsky, 2018). However, with others, communication about boundaries must be more direct. In all cases, when a boundary is crossed, feedback must be given that it's not OK, or anger and resentment will occur. A boundary is worthless if it is not enforced by feedback and consequences (Martin, 2018b).

"When you feel yourself becoming angry, resentful, or exhausted, pay attention to where you haven't set a healthy boundary."

—Crystal Andrus

For example, one professional boundary might be to avoid sharing your work-related frustrations with coworkers. Every person in authority needs to vent and talk to someone safe about the challenges of the job—and get an outsider's take on some of the human resource issues that are a part of any management position. But this person should not be a subordinate. Preferably, it wouldn't even be someone who works in the same organization.

Social media is also not a safe place for venting, even though it may feel safer than talking directly to colleagues at work. Privacy on the internet is an illusion, even if you have been careful not to initiate or accept a friend request from an employee. I'm always amazed what colleagues post on the internet about their job, their boss, or troubles they're experiencing at work. I don't care how private you think your post is, once someone shares it, the whole world has access to what you said.

In addition, it may be necessary to create a boundary in terms of allowing others to have opinions different from yours, even if you believe their views are wrong. Martin (2018b) notes that healthy emotional boundaries mean you value your own feelings and needs, and you're not responsible for how others feel or behave. Boundaries allow you to let go of worrying about how others feel and place accountability squarely with the individual.

> ## "Boundaries let people know that you respect yourself."
> —Beate Chelette

"For better or for worse, Facebook, Twitter and Instagram have broken down a lot of professional boundaries. Before social media, you probably didn't know much about your employees' social lives. Now, however, if you're friends with them on Facebook, you can see updates about everything from what they ate for dinner last night to the adorable things their kids did over the weekend."

—Robert Half

Similarly, Reilly (2017) asserts that sometimes we want and expect those close to us to act in a specific way and to support us. When they don't, we feel hurt. But when we let go of those expectations by respecting that everyone needs boundaries, relationships cannot only be salvaged but also strengthened.

Lancer (2016) concurs, noting that healthy boundaries prevent you from giving advice and blaming or accepting blame. They also protect you from feeling guilty for someone else's negative feelings or problems and taking other people's comments personally. When you overreact to or personalize the feelings or actions of others, you are demonstrating weak emotional boundaries. Healthy emotional boundaries require clear internal boundaries—knowing how you feel and what responsibilities you have to yourself and others.

Another professional boundary is separating work time from family or personal time. Perfectly balancing life's components is impossible. Instead, we should try to be flexible about what we need to focus on at a specific point in time.

For example, far too many people run themselves into the ground—mentally and physically—to meet other people's needs. Being afraid to say no to others can lead to a "spiral of shame," Chun (2018) says, because your inner voice may tell you that you are missing out, you are not good enough, or you are letting others or yourself down. But the truth is, saying no simply means that what you've been asked to do doesn't align with your priorities or that something else is more important to do at the time. There is no need to overexplain or apologize for saying no. We all have the right to determine what we want to do and what we don't want to do.

In fact, self-care is an often-neglected priority for leaders. It is OK to put yourself first at times. Leaders should seek time off on a regular basis to meet personal needs, seek recreation, form relationships outside the work setting, and have fun. For example, I am an avid duplicate bridge player. My friends at the bridge club know little about my professional life, and that is an intentional boundary I have created.

Leaders should also seek out friends and family for emotional support, guidance, and renewal. In addition, a proper diet and exercise are important to maintain both physical and emotional health. Spirituality may also be important in self-care. Leaders should remember that there is life outside of work, and that time should be relished and protected.

Creating space between personal and professional relationships is an important boundary for managers. Without that space, a manager's formal authority to direct others may be questioned or lost. Half (2015) notes that even just a decade ago, many managers avoided get-togethers outside of work, and friendships at work were considered off-limits. Today, more casual relationships between bosses and employees have become part of a larger

"Boundaries aren't about trying to control someone or make them change. Boundaries are about establishing how you want to be treated, self-preservation in a chaotic or dangerous environment, and a path to healthy relationships."

—Sharon Martin (2018a)

transformation of the workplace. Most experts now believe that socializing outside the workplace can help leaders build trust with their team and improve morale. Indeed, most employees enjoy getting to know their boss a little bit better on a personal level, and employees with a strong connection to their managers are more likely to work longer hours and be loyal to the company (All Business, 2019).

In addition, as a boss, having friendships with your employees allows you to have a strong, positive relationship with them. It also helps you understand what motivates them because you learn about their families, interests, and goals in life (All Business, 2019).

The reality is, friendships and social relationships are very common between leaders and employees because we spend so much time at work. The problem is that people can become confused about their relationship with their boss. In addition, workers pay attention to whom their leader has lunch with or interacts with socially. And no matter how hard you try to be impartial, some will always believe that the individuals you have a personal friendship with receive special favors or consideration.

I found this to be the case when I was Director of a School of Nursing. When faculty received teaching assignments they wanted, they perceived the assignment process to be fair. When the same faculty were asked to teach courses they didn't prefer, they often suggested that assignments had been based on friendship.

Ironically, a recent study showed that employers are more likely to skip over their friends to reward employees they're not close to in an effort to avoid appearing biased (Jones, 2018). That was the case even if the manager's friend was slightly more deserving. Thus, perceptions of bias can occur both ways, and the only way to avoid this risk is to avoid the conflict of interest entirely.

If you decide to cross the friendship line, make sure to clarify the boundaries of the relationship. For example, as the boss, you will still be tasked with their performance reviews and performance problems. Your friends should know that, if their behavior is not up to par or is negatively impacting employee morale, work schedules, or work culture, you will be their employer first and their friend second (All Business, 2019). This does not mean that putting on your "boss hat" when it is needed will be appreciated at the time—or that your forewarning will be remembered. In addition, some lines should never be crossed, such as sharing information about one employee with another if there is no official need to know.

Surprisingly, leadership and management can be lonely enterprises at times. Having appropriate personal and professional boundaries, however, allows the leader to consistently do the right thing. This comes only from clarity about personal values and what the leadership role should be.

"As we look ahead into the next century, leaders will be those who empower others."

—Bill Gates

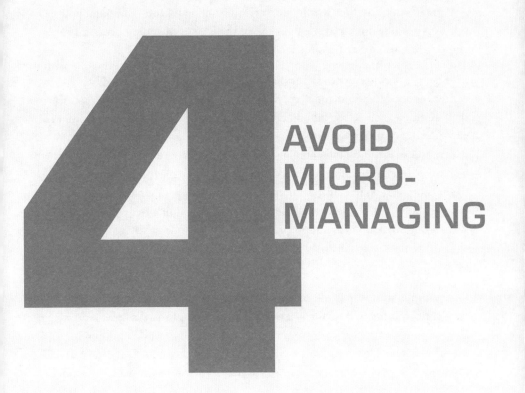

4 AVOID MICRO-MANAGING

Another strategy for creating positive work cultures is to avoid micromanaging. In other words, stop creating so many rules, surround yourself with good people, and then get out of the way of the employees you've empowered, whenever possible!

Micromanagement refers to situations where managers feel the need to control every decision made and every task to be completed. In other words, they immerse themselves fully in tasks that are to be accomplished by others and dictate every step to be taken. In addition, they constantly experience frustration with what they perceive as substandard work because no one can live up to their expectations. Indeed, "nothing is too insignificant, too mundane, and even too irrelevant to bypass a micromanager's wrath" (Reuter, 2018, para. 1). While being sure that employees are doing the right thing and getting work done are appropriate management tasks, paying attention to and attempting to control even irrelevant details are signs of micromanagement.

For example, most experienced nurses working in a hospital have a beginning shift routine that includes performing baseline physical assessments, checking medications to be given, reviewing critical lab work, and looking for new orders. The order in which these tasks are accomplished often varies, depending on patient needs or nurse preference. A micromanager would want all nurses to do the tasks in the manager's preferred order and manner and then would constantly check to make sure that happened.

Micromanagement, then, is the ultimate controlling management style. "It's demoralizing and counter-intuitive, as the desire for control to make sure everything goes to plan only creates more problems in the long-term" (Mulholland, 2018, para. 4). Magnuson (2017) agrees, noting that employees' self-motivation, initiative, and creativity plummet under the control of a micromanager. That's because micromanagement stifles creative thinking and demotivates employees who want to learn and demonstrate independent thought or action. Employees who are micromanaged typically feel that their boss does not trust them.

In addition, it is difficult to perform well and be innovative when someone constantly checks on you and scrutinizes every detail of your work. In fact, a study published in the *Journal of Experimental Psychology* found that people who believe they are being watched perform at a lower level because "choking under pressure" can be triggered by "explicitly monitoring" (Molloy, 2017, para. 5).

I can remember feeling like I had to walk on eggshells when I worked for a micromanager. She needed nearly constant updates on delegated tasks and was often critical of what I accomplished. She often redid tasks, or a portion of them, to meet her standards or be sure they were done "the right way." After a time, I just stopped trying because I knew it would never be good enough. Indeed, when managers believe their team can't be trusted to do a good job, the team often begins to believe it as well. Micromanagement is a sure way to ensure your team won't reach its full potential.

Ironically, micromanaging is generally an outgrowth of inexperience or insecurity, not a demonstration of competence or expertise on the part of the leader. Micromanagers typically fear that, if their employees fail, they will look like a failure as well. As a result, they tightly guard new opportunities for growth and innovation and set goals for workers that are based on what is safe, not on individual potential.

Micromanagement is also exhausting. Looking over so many shoulders every day can lead to burning out and hating your job because the energy burned by micromanaging will ignite that wick faster than anything. In addition, as you "flame out," you'll likely take your staff with you. Indeed, a study by Harry Chambers (as cited in Coolman, n.d.), author of *My Way or the Highway: The Micromanagement Survival Guide*, found that 71% of nonmanagers said micromanagement had interfered with their job performance, and 85% said it had damaged their morale. Another study by Accountemps (as cited in Molloy, 2017) showed similar findings, in that nearly 70% of workers said micromanagement had decreased their morale.

Finally, micromanagement slows down work. In a study of companies in Europe and the United States, Boston Consulting Group (as cited in Molloy, 2017) found that, from 2012 to 2017, the number of procedures, vertical layers, interface structures, coordination bodies, and decision approvals needed has increased by up to 350% in some organizations. The result? Progress in completing projects or goals has slowed or ground to a halt completely.

"Micromanagement will eventually lead to a massive breakdown of trust. Your staff will no longer see you as a manager, but a despot whose only desire is to wall up its staff until the only thing they see is the job."

—Jack Wallen

When micromanagement is the result of a rigidly hierarchical culture, managers themselves may be micromanaged, and these effects can filter down throughout the organization.

What are the solutions to micromanagement? One solution is *macromanagement*, the opposite of micromanagement (Britcher, 2018). Macromanagers set clear expectations and define how performance will be measured but welcome input and are willing to tweak the process. Macromanagement, then, is about initiating dialogue about assignments and asking open-ended questions that convey interest, accountability, and autonomy about how assignments might be carried out.

The first step in macromanagement is selecting the right person to carry out a task. It is important to identify which individuals can complete a job in terms of capability and time to do so. In addition, leaders should look for opportunities to stretch capable employees who want opportunities to learn and grow and innovative employees who are willing to take risks.

It is also important that the person who is assigned a task considers the task important. This does not mean that skill and expertise are not needed. Managers should always ask individuals if they can complete delegated tasks and validate this by direct observation.

After the project has been assigned, leaders should ask employees to describe the desired outcome in their own words. This confirms there is a shared understanding of the assignment to be completed and lets employees highlight the unique strengths or skills they have to accomplish the work.

Macromanagement also requires setting clear expectations regarding the assigned task (Britcher, 2018). Expected deliverables should always be clearly communicated as should any limitations, boundaries, or qualifications that are being imposed on the task. Employees must be given enough information to know what the desired product should be, but they should have an appropriate degree of autonomy in deciding how the work will be accomplished. It is important to give employees permission to be creative in how they accomplish the task. Westfall (2019, para. 6) notes, "In the industrial production model (think Henry Ford), it was important for everyone on the assembly line to perform the same task with the same tools the same way. In the modern work environment, away from the assembly line, there are many paths to the same destination."

Leaders must also make sure they have delegated the authority and responsibility necessary to complete the assigned task. Stoker (2018) agrees, noting that leaders should ask employees what they need to complete their projects on time, including additional manpower, time, money, equipment, or training. Nothing is more frustrating to creative and productive employees than not having the resources or authority they need to carry out a well-developed plan. Yet, this transfer of power is one of the most difficult tasks for micromanagers.

"Never tell people how to do things. Tell them what to do and they will surprise you with their ingenuity."

—George S. Patton

The next step in macromanagement is to establish clear milestones for task completion, including a timeline, and to check in with employees regularly—weekly or biweekly—to make sure they are making progress. That way, there will be time to readjust if the employee needs further direction or encounters unexpected obstacles. It is important, though, to have reasonable expectations of what the selected individual can do with the time and resources available.

In addition, leaders should expect that employees will encounter challenges and obstacles when asked to perform new or difficult tasks. Being a role model and a resource, however, doesn't mean stepping in to solve those problems the minute an employee encounters them. Instead, the leader's role is to answer questions about the task or clarify desired outcomes as necessary. It could also be simply offering encouragement, being a sounding board, acknowledging efforts, or helping identify possible solutions to the problems.

Leaders must also make sure to express appreciation to employees when they make progress in completing a task. When leaders focus on what's working well, they reduce anxieties and invite participation (Britcher, 2018). They also create a shared experience and an even stronger foundation on which to grow, experiment, or try new things.

Finally, taking back a delegated task should be a leader's last resort because this action fosters a sense of failure in the employee. It's so easy to fall into the trap of "my way is the best way" or "I know best." Delegation is useless if the manager is unwilling to allow divergence in problem-solving and thus redoes the work that has been delegated. If this happens, the task likely should not have been delegated in the first place.

"Micromanaging erodes people's confidence, making them overly dependent on their leaders. Well-meaning leaders inadvertently sabotage their teams by rushing to the rescue and offering too much help. A leader needs to balance assistance with wu wei*, backing off long enough to let people learn from their mistakes and develop competence."

—Diane Dreher

*In Chinese, wu wei means doing nothing.

"Problems keep mounting so fast that we find ourselves taking shortcuts to temporarily alleviate the tension points—so we can move onto the next problem. In the process, we fail to solve the core of each problem we are dealt; thus we continuously get caught in the trap of a never-ending cycle that makes it difficult to find any real resolutions."

—Glenn Llopis

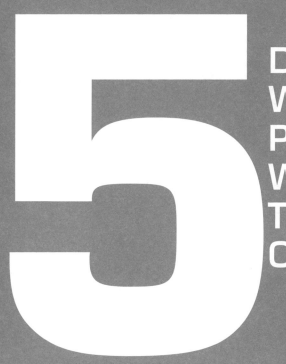

5

**DEAL
WITH
PROBLEMS
WHEN
THEY
OCCUR**

Another leadership strategy for creating a positive work culture is to deal with problems as soon as they occur. The road to both life and success is paved with obstacles and difficulties. All leaders encounter problems as well as successes. Indeed, many leaders say they spend as much time in coming up with workarounds and repairing damage as they do in attaining organizational goals.

Unfortunately, leaders sometimes procrastinate solving important problems. To *procrastinate* means to put off something until a future time, to postpone, or to delay needlessly. Procrastination in solving a problem is justified only if another issue is of greater importance at that moment. It should not be used to avoid a task that is overwhelming or unpleasant. Workers look to their leaders to fix problems and get discouraged when they see problems go unaddressed.

Indeed, problem-solving is a big part of what leaders do. One goal for us as leaders is to minimize the occurrence of problems, which means we must be courageous enough to tackle them head-on before circumstances force our hand. And we must be resilient in our quest to create and sustain momentum for the organization and people we serve.

"Avoid letting problems linger. Addressing issues as they occur is a much better strategy than waiting for things to get better and work themselves out. Employees get discouraged when they see problems go unaddressed. It may take more time to handle a problem right away and it may be unpleasant, but it is much better than what you'll have to face if you allow it to fester."

—Kate McFarlin

For example, a new faculty member was hired to teach in my School of Nursing. Her resume was impressive, she had extensive clinical experience, and she was articulate in her hiring interviews. The problem was that she couldn't teach. Early student feedback suggested that her lectures were poorly organized, she lacked essential skills in the clinical setting, she did not provide timely or meaningful feedback, and she sometimes missed classes without notifying students. When the faculty member was confronted with these concerns, she explained away most as coming from a few disgruntled students. The complaints, however, eventually became a pattern that could not be ignored. Despite extensive coaching and mentoring, that faculty member was not successful in the role, and her position was terminated. Keeping her in hope that someday the situation would change would have been a disservice both to students and the faculty member, who certainly would not have been successful in achieving tenure and promotion.

Managers face problems almost every day, and the variety of problems is nearly endless. One common problem is interprofessional conflict. Conflict can result anytime two or more people have differences in ideas, values, or feelings. Conflict is part of life. So is dealing with difficult people or with those who have different expectations, needs, or wants than we do. When these relationships matter or when the issue at debate is important, spending time and effort to resolve differences makes sense because new collaborations—or at least an appreciation of divergent opinions—often results (Huston, 2018).

Conflict, then, should be an expected occurrence in all organizations. As such, it can disrupt working relationships and result in lower productivity if not managed appropriately. It is imperative that leaders identify the origin of conflicts when they first occur and intervene as necessary to promote cooperative, if not collaborative, conflict resolution.

If conflict occurs because workers are unwilling to follow rules or established policies and procedures—or are unable to perform duties adequately despite assistance and encouragement—the leader has an obligation to take disciplinary action, no matter how unpleasant. It can be difficult, though, to determine the appropriate level of discipline needed. Inappropriate discipline (too much or too little) can undermine the morale of the whole team and become more destructive than constructive.

To avoid this, discipline is generally administered using a model that progresses from a verbal warning to a written warning, suspension, and termination. Except in limited circumstances, employees should be given the opportunity to correct problems. If it becomes apparent, however, that a progressive disciplinary approach has failed, and necessary behavior change has not occurred, managers may need to terminate the employee.

Delay in addressing the problem only exacerbates such situations. The disenchantment of a single employee can spread, affecting employees who are otherwise satisfied and highly valued. When someone is not performing well, everyone knows it. And when management refuses to act, employees may perceive that their leaders lack the resolve necessary to make the organization successful.

Another common type of conflict in the work setting is interpersonal conflict between employees. When this occurs, the leader needs to think carefully about how best to intervene. Many times, team members inappropriately expect a manager to solve their interpersonal conflicts. The manager who does this has little to gain and a lot to lose. In most cases, leaders should urge subordinates to try to resolve their own conflicts before intervening.

When that doesn't work, leaders can and should act as a neutral third party to help workers overcome the hurdle of not listening to each other or to bring issues to the forefront. This only works, though, if all parties are motivated to solve the problem and if differences do not exist in their status or power. If the conflict involves multiple parties and highly charged emotions, the manager may find that outside experts can help facilitate communication and bring issues to the forefront.

Interpersonal conflicts between managers and workers are also likely to occur. Those in charge do not have to like everyone who works for them, as long as some degree of tolerance and mutual respect is maintained. Some workers, however, continuously push boundaries and create unpleasant work environments. For example, I worked for decades with a rude, outspoken faculty member who bullied her way through most faculty meetings, interrupting continuously and often insulting others in attendance. Efforts to

"Seemingly inconsequential acts of bad behavior can spread through your organization like the flu, taking a financial and emotional toll if left unchecked."

—Christine Pearson

confront her bullying behavior were limited because most of the faculty, including the dean, were afraid of her.

Similarly, I had a student who made a point of repeatedly yawning and stretching very loudly during class to show that he was bored. A smug smile and wave to his classmates always followed this behavior. This passive–aggressive behavior was generally met with a few giggles from classmates, subtly encouraging this behavior to continue. One day, I stopped in the middle of my lecture and directedly asked the student if he was bored and wanted to leave. He really wanted to say yes but lacked the courage to do so. The direct confrontation stopped the behavior almost completely.

When should you step back or ignore unruly behavior, and when is it worthy of intervention? It depends on how important the issue is. If only your ego has been damaged, it may not be worth the fight (Huston, 2018). With the passive–aggressive student in my classroom, the most appropriate response was to confront him, in front of other students, with the intent of his message. The student then had to immediately confirm what the intent of his behavior was or lose credibility in front of his peers. Either way, he lost the power of plausible deniability.

In the case of the bullying faculty member, confrontation was also needed. (Civility is addressed fully in Chapter 2.) Attempting to rationally reason with bullies, however, does not always work. With some bad behavior,

"Silence is always a go-to strategy for passive—aggressors and it's not hard to see why. It says nothing at all and yet says volumes. It ostensibly avoids a conflict but in fact provokes one—with the very lack of communication serving as a taunt and a goad. It's thus passive, and yet, um, aggressive."

—Jeffrey Kluger

especially if it has minimal impact on others, it may be appropriate to simply remain calm, walk away, and not react. Many people behave in obnoxious ways to get attention, and the behavior may diminish if they don't receive reinforcement (Huston, 2018). You can't always control the behavior of others, but you *can* control your response and learn to react in a way that allows you to move forward.

Beard, McGinn, and Edmondson (2018) suggest, however, that framing bad behavior as tolerable—or even worse, as acceptable—is problematic because all you can do is "tell the person, well that's really bad and not working, or stay silent. Those are your only two options. And neither one of them works very well" (para. 74). So, if the short- or long-term results of not addressing a conflict have significant, negative consequences for you or others, addressing the situation is imperative.

Another problem that leaders face in the workplace occurs when teams don't work well together to achieve agreed-upon goals. Team members who disconnect become nonfunctional. Often, this occurs because of communication breakdowns. When facing a dysfunctional team, leaders must diagnose the problem and take immediate corrective action to avoid the problem spreading throughout the organization. Otherwise, staff can split into multiple groups, all at odds with each other. These problems can eliminate the positive work culture you have been carefully cultivating.

"Major hurdles are disheartening, and they're often unavoidable. But the way you engage with and think about problems directly influences your ability to solve them."

—Daniel Marlin

"A team without trust isn't really a team: it's just a group of individuals, working together, often making disappointing progress."

–Mind Tools

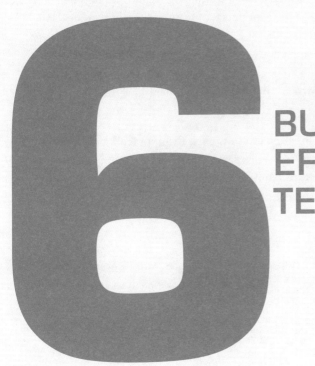

6

BUILD EFFECTIVE TEAMS

Another strategy crucial for positive work cultures is team-building. People in every workplace talk about the importance of building teams, but many don't understand the experience of teamwork or how to develop effective teams. The reality is that it is difficult to build effective organizational teams because organizations are made up of individuals with different worldviews, values, fears, and confidence levels. In addition, while employees may understand how their job fits within the hierarchy, they may not have internalized being a part of a larger team.

Belonging to a team, in the broadest sense, is a result of feeling part of something larger than yourself. For example, a basketball team may be composed of technically excellent players, but if those players can't learn to merge their skills, communicate well, and work together to achieve a common goal (winning the game), their individual skill levels become almost immaterial.

A similar analogy can be made for a rapid response team responding to a cardiac event. If the person doing cardiac compressions doesn't work closely with the respiratory therapist providing artificial ventilation or the pharmacist administering medications or the physician observing the cardiac monitor, the likelihood of successful patient resuscitation declines dramatically.

Similarly, employees in an organization must work collectively to achieve the organization's mission and vision rather than a specific task or goal. For example, nursing faculty members may focus heavily on developing content for the specialty area they are teaching but fail to recognize that this content must fit into an orderly and well-developed curriculum that meets desired end-of-program learning outcomes. The leader's role is to blend individuals with different talents, strengths, and motivations into a team to accomplish organizational goals.

Fortunately, most employees want to be part of something bigger than themselves. "They no longer work for companies just to have the company name on their resume. Employees, particularly the younger generations, want to know *why* they are doing what they are doing. It is not enough to just know how, they want to know the impact of their efforts. They want to feel intimately connected to the goal and to their part in reaching that goal" (Work Points Play, n.d., para. 2).

Thus, one of the first things leaders must do to create effective teams is to establish relationships with team members. Edmonds (2018) agrees, noting the importance of leaders regularly connecting with people at all levels in the organization. Leaders who take the time to learn the names of their employees and what their passions are send a message that the organization cares about their personal well-being.

A hospital CEO at one of my earliest nursing jobs would walk the halls every day, stopping to visit with patients and employees. He knew virtually every employee's name and often knew enough about the employee's family or interests to engage in a meaningful personal conversation. Initially, I wondered why he did this, or if he just had a lot of extra time on his hands, but I now realize what an incredible leader he was. Employees worked harder because they didn't want to disappoint him, and I, like almost everyone else, came to look forward to his daily check-in because it made me feel valued and appreciated.

Stoker (2018) agrees, noting that employees want to work for "super humans," not "superhumans." Super humans take an interest in those around them and have a knack for connecting with people—no matter who they are. They speak to individual employees by name and ask how they are doing so that staff members feel their boss has their best interests at heart.

For example, another CEO I worked with would occasionally come in during night shift to help serve meals in the cafeteria. He did this so that he could form relationships with staff who sometimes felt invisible or forgotten. These types of interactions build loyalty and trust. But building genuine, extensive relationships takes time.

"It's a lot easier to get behind a leader who is in the trenches with you. Show your team that you can roll up your sleeves and help get things done. Understanding what your team does and how hard they work will help develop respect. Also remember that honesty leads to credibility. If you realize you've messed up, don't be afraid to say so."

—John Pettit

It also requires some vulnerability on the part of leaders. That means being willing to share mistakes they have made or expertise they may lack. For example, some leaders openly share stories about successes and failures they have experienced in their lives to help followers avoid making the same mistakes and to create a sense of camaraderie. When leaders share these stories, employees see them both as humble and authentic. It also builds trust and may open lines of communication that become more important over time.

Remember, the most effective leaders build their teams based on trust and loyalty, rather than fear or the power of their positions. Leaders, then, must have a propensity to trust others, and they must go first in extending that trust. Covey (2019, para. 18) notes that this is "not a blind trust without expectations and accountability, but rather a 'smart trust' with clear expectations and strong accountability built into the process."

Covey (2019) also suggests that the trust between leaders and their teams is born from both character and competence. Character includes integrity, motive, and intent with people. "When you consistently do the right thing whether you feel like it or not, when your actions match your words, and when you support your team in every situation, you give people evidence of your character" (Daskal, n.d., para. 3).

"When trust is low, in a company or in a relationship, it places a hidden 'tax' on every transaction: every communication, every interaction, every strategy, every decision is taxed, bringing speed down and sending costs up. My experience is that significant distrust doubles the cost of doing business and triples the time it takes to get things done."

—Stephen M. R. Covey

Competence includes your capabilities, skills, results, and track record. It also includes knowing what you don't know. "It's important that you know what you're doing—and when you don't know something, that you have the fortitude to admit it" (Daskal, n.d., para. 6). Both dimensions are vital to build trust between leaders and followers.

Leaders must also encourage trust and cooperation among members of the team because those relationships are every bit as important as those the leader establishes with them. In fact, according to a 2017 Employee Engagement Report, what employees love most about their jobs is their coworkers (Reynolds, 2017). Indeed, Davis (2018) notes that even if you have the "right people on the bus" (the right talent), it's the nature of the relationships among those people—the work culture—that really creates a competitive advantage for a team or organization. Work culture often makes or breaks the success and effectiveness of an organization.

Indeed, Figliuolo (2018) suggests that chemistry and trust among team members are what differentiate a regular team from a high-performing team. These intangibles are critical elements of team-building, but developing these resilient bonds is not easy because leaders must understand different personalities and create shared beliefs. Leaders, then, must set aside adequate time and resources to help employees know and understand each other.

In addition, as the team begins to take shape, leaders should pay close attention to the ways in which team members work together and take steps to improve communication, cooperation, trust, and respect in those relationships. How team members feel about their coworkers can affect how effectively a team works together.

Facilitating communication is also important. Leaders must be effective communicators themselves and role-model excellent communication skills to team members. Indeed, communication is a critical factor in successful teamwork. Scott (2019) concurs, noting that communication and team-building are intertwined because team-building activities encourage trust, cooperation, and communication within a group, and improving communication enhances how workers interact with one another.

For example, some organizations encourage team members to complete self-assessment tools that identify personal strengths, predominant leadership styles, and personality or psychological preferences. Teams are then encouraged to share results with each other so that members not only get to know each other better but also better understand each other's strengths and weaknesses in accomplishing shared goals.

> ## "With the right leadership, the entire team makes the climb."
> —Chris Westfall

Leaders must also communicate what is expected of each team member. Effective leaders listen to what team members say about each other and about the team in a nonjudgmental manner. If team members share a concern, steps should be taken to resolve the issue as quickly as possible and to keep the team informed regarding the resolution.

In addition, it is critical to keep people up to speed on what is going on, even when times are tough. "If you don't, the hall chatter begins and the rumor mill becomes toxic" (Barter, 2017, para. 8). People are the most important asset in an organization. "When there is little to no transparency, people wonder what you are hiding and start to question your key decisions and actions" (Barter, 2017, para. 8).

Hoff (2018) also notes that ongoing communication is essential among team members. When possible, leaders should schedule brief weekly meetings to make sure team members are on board with priorities and where their efforts should be focused. These meetings are also a good time to recognize the progress the team has made. In addition, leaders should use two-way feedback to promote continued improvement, upward progress—and ultimately, better performance.

Cummings (2013) refers to trust, communication, and leadership as the three-legged stool of modern organizations. It is intentional that communication falls between trust and leadership because communication is the thread that enables leaders to create a culture of trust within their organization. Once trust is established, leaders can achieve their goals more effectively with the support of their team.

"You can have a compelling vision, rock-solid strategy, excellent communication skills, innovative insight, and a skilled team, but if people don't trust you, you will never get the results you want."

—David Horsager

"Stress and anxiety at work have less to do with the work we do and more to do with weak management and leadership."

—Simon Sinek

7

REDUCE
WORKPLACE
STRESS

Another strategy for creating positive work cultures is to reduce workplace stress. The American Institute of Stress (n.d.) cites numerous studies showing that job stress is far and away the major source of stress for American adults and that it has escalated progressively over the past few decades. Lipman (2019) agrees, noting that work is inherently stressful. In addition, recent survey results showed 66% of respondents had lost sleep due to work-related stress, 16% had quit a job because stress had become too overwhelming, and 76% said workplace stress had a negative impact on their personal relationships. The survey also indicated that overall employee stress levels had risen nearly 20% in three decades.

Research data suggests the problem may be even worse in nursing. A recent study revealed that an overwhelming 92% of nurses experience moderate to very high stress levels (Advance Staff, 2018). This finding supports another study showing nearly half of nurses under 30 years old—and 40% of those over 40—are experiencing burnout (Advance Staff, 2018). As the industry continues its shift toward value-based care and the demand for nurses intensifies, managers need to identify the causes of this stress and find ways to give nurses the support they need.

"**Depression is an epidemic in nursing, but no one will talk about it. According to the Robert Wood Johnson Foundation Interdisciplinary Nursing Quality Research Initiative (INQRI), nurses experience clinical depression at twice the rate of the general public. Depression affects 9% of everyday citizens, but 18% of nurses experience symptoms of depression.**"

—Lynda Lampert

What are the biggest causes of stress at work? There are many, but the severity of job stress typically depends on the demands being made and the sense of control an individual has in dealing with them. Stress, however, is a highly personalized phenomenon. Some people thrive in the fast lane—having to perform multiple things simultaneously, which would overwhelm most people. Their stress level may be fairly low if they perceive they are in control. Other employees, with far lower workloads, feel stressed much of the time. Stress levels, then, can vary widely, even in identical situations.

This suggests that to create a positive work culture, managers must be attentive to work demands and also to assuring that workers feel some sense of control over their working conditions. For example, according to a recent survey by Harris Interactive (as cited in ICA Notes, 2018), 48% of workers report having unreasonable deadlines. Managers, then, must be sure that assigned workloads are reasonable. The reality is that employees sometimes fail simply because the workload was too great to be reasonably accomplished, not because they lacked the skills to do the job. They were set up for failure due to unrealistic expectations.

"As their role expands from the bedside to the waiting room to the board room, nurses are busier than ever and increasingly stressed. Beyond providing direct medical care, nurses are also an educational resource, an advocate for patient needs, and a source of comfort. Combined, these factors are contributing to soaring stress levels and burnout."

—Advance Staff

We often see this with new nurse graduates. There are still differences between expectations in the academic and work world, and most new graduates need time to learn the complexities of the professional nursing role. Sometimes, coworkers lack patience during the new graduate nurse's journey. Indeed, 90% of new graduate nurses report bullying from other nurses (Thompson, 2019).

I still remember how scary it was to be a new graduate. Like most new graduates, I suffered a bit from "imposter syndrome." Although I had good grades, I wondered if my instructors knew how uncertain I felt about my skills and my ability to work independently. There was a big learning curve in that transition from academe to practice, especially that first year after graduation. I would often get to the end of the day and recall something critical I should have done but forgot because I was so overwhelmed by everything I had to remember. It would have been even more overwhelming if my coworkers had not been supportive and encouraging.

Yazdi (2019, para. 10) shares similar thoughts in her tips to nurses:

> Your situation today will not be your situation forever! Back when I started my nursing career, I fell into a strange depression that came from a place of starting a career I didn't know if I really liked, working nights, and feeling really alone and incompetent to boot. Now looking back (that was only a handful of years ago)

> I realize that those first few years were just a small speck on the
> timeline of my life. I did my due diligence of gaining my experi-
> ence … and although I still get quite frustrated with the nature of
> the job, I know better than to feel like there is no end in sight.

This need for new graduates to "hit the ground running" has manifested
into a phenomenon known as *reality* or *transition shock*. The fear of making a
mistake becomes absolutely crippling to a new graduate's confidence and self-
image. It's the fear that is crippling, not the actual lack of knowledge.

Nurse residencies are one bridge to this problem. These programs focus
on imparting preliminary experience, job expectations, and overall self-
confidence to new nursing graduates prior to entering their first job. The
leadership and communication skills these new graduates attain as a result
of participation in the nurse residency reduce work stress as well as turnover
rates. Assigning experienced mentors and preceptors to new graduates is another possible solution because they can provide one-on-one support in terms
of encouragement, role-modeling, and direct competency improvement.

But even the most supportive work environment won't help if workload
demands are unreasonable. We continue to see staff nurses with extraordinary workloads, even though a rapidly growing body of literature shows that
having fewer RNs in the staffing mix and an increased workload are linked to

negative patient outcomes, including falls and medication errors. As a result, many nurses work longer shifts or are forced to work overtime, and patients are sicker than ever.

In addition, nursing is both physically and emotionally demanding. Hours are long; fatigue related to the physical demands of moving constantly, lifting, and bending is common; and shift work can lead to unhealthy imbalances in circadian rhythms. Caregiving can also be emotionally draining for the nurse, who is often challenged to meet the differing expectations of the employer, patient, family, professional boards, and self. *Compassion fatigue* refers to the weariness that develops from caring for individuals when caregivers feel saddened that they cannot change the situation and give of themselves in the hope of relieving pain or suffering in the patient (Wojciechowski, 2018).

Karen Whitehead (as cited in Wojciechowski, 2018) notes that anyone who is empathetic and works in a caregiving role is "at risk for developing compassion fatigue and increased caregiver stress, which affects emotional health. Nurses who over-identify with patients and blur boundaries, as well as nurses with personal trauma histories, poor social support, isolated working conditions, or a previous history of unmanaged anxiety are at greater risk" (para. 5).

Another source of stress in workplaces is constant change. Many organizations today are either considering or enacting a transformation of some type. Thus, "change is the new normal" has become a reality, and most organizations feel like they can't be reinvented fast enough.

Just look back at how healthcare has changed in the past decade—healthcare reform, accountable care organizations, reimbursement based on quality not on volume, electronic health records, computerized provider order entry, and clinical decision support. In addition, genetics and genomics have changed the focus of healthcare from treating illness to treating diseases, through precision medicine, that people have an increased risk of developing. All these changes have reduced a sense of control in the workplace.

People like feeling safe, comfortable, and in control of their environment. When work is in a constant state of flux, workers feel unsettled and unsure of themselves. The leader's role is to make sure that change for the sake of change doesn't happen. Change needs to occur for a good reason, and workers need to understand how the change will make things better and, specifically, how it will impact them.

Leaders also must act as role models during the change process. When leaders are stressed and impart a sense of things being out of control, followers quickly adopt the same attitude. In fact, attitude is everything. Rather than viewing change as a threat, leaders need to embrace it and actively role-model this for staff. Then they need to help staff members do the same.

Leaders also must show that they personally can find some balance between change and stability in their lives. This feeling of control is probably the most important trait for thriving in a changing environment. Leaders need to recognize their own stress signals during change and take appropriate steps when the stress level rises too high.

Finally, leaders must look for ways to empower workers. To empower means to enable, develop, or allow. One way leaders can empower subordinates is by delegating assignments to provide learning opportunities and allowing them to share in the satisfaction derived from achievement. Another strategy is to assist staff members in building their personal power base. This can be accomplished by showing subordinates how their personal, expert, and referent power can be expanded.

For example, Marquis and Huston (2020) note that personal power can be increased by being a team player, being flexible, showing a genuine interest in and support of others, and developing a voice within the organization.

Expert power increases as an individual gains knowledge, expertise, or experience. Having knowledge and skill that others lack can greatly augment a person's power base. Thus, returning to school for further education or achieving specialty certification can increase one's expert power.

Finally, an individual gains referent power when others identify with the person—or with what that person symbolizes. Thus, having a broad vision and presenting a powerful picture to others can build referent power.

Empowerment also occurs when workers are involved in planning and implementing change—and when workers believe that they have some input in what is about to happen and some control over the environment in which they will work in the future. Leaders should never get so excited, however, about things they want *others* to do that they lose sight of what *they* want to do.

> ## "The empowerment of staff is a hallmark of transformational leadership."
> —Bessie Marquis & Carol Huston

"People want to know they matter and they want to be treated as people. That's the new talent contract."

—Pamela Stroko

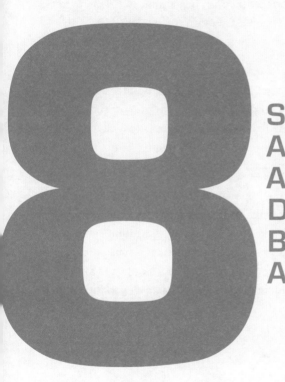

8

**SHOW
APPRECIATION
AND REWARD
DESIRED
BEHAVIOR
APPROPRIATELY**

Another strategy for creating a positive work culture is to show appreciation to employees. This appreciation must be genuine and somewhat individual in nature because most people are motivated and engaged only when they feel truly appreciated in a way that is both accurate and personal (Craemer, 2018).

Indeed, "the idea that it's not personal, it's 'just business' is a notion from a past time" (Naseer, n.d., para. 23). Today's workers want greater connection with those in charge—not only feedback about their performance but also conversations that make them feel that what they do matters and that their employers care about their ability to succeed.

In other words, employees want the opportunity to grow, learn, and make a difference, and they want to know that their manager is aware of their unique contributions when they make these efforts. These moments of connection, of conversing with those you lead, help engender a sense of meaning and purpose within your team. In addition, the deciding factor for why people stay at a job or look elsewhere often has to do with the relationship they have with their manager.

"Brains, like hearts, go where they are appreciated."

—Robert McNamara, former U.S. Secretary of Defense

I have worked extraordinarily hard, sometimes without reimbursement, for leaders and organizations when I felt appreciated. The converse is true as well. When I am made to feel inconsequential, my motivation to do my best declines.

What, then, are the best ways to show appreciation to employees? Believe it or not, it's not always monetary, although money is a strong motivator for many people. Other ways organizations can show appreciation and recognition include promotions, new titles or job responsibilities, or even a plaque to hang on the wall. But which strategy is most effective? It depends. In fact, what motivates one individual or group may not be valued by another.

Organizations must recognize and reward employees in a way that means something to them. Giving gift cards to all employees at Christmas or standardized retirement gifts—while important—are not enough. Neither are annual merit raises because most employees view them as a universal "given." Giving employees an "ugly sweater" is awesome if they want an ugly sweater or live someplace where they can use a sweater in general (Lauby, 2019). Thus, incentives are powerful only if the individual or group places importance on the reward.

In addition, the value of some incentives can change over time and in different situations (Cherry, 2019a). Leaders must attempt to understand the values of the different teams they work with and the cultures they work in and try to create recognition programs that meet those values.

> "Appreciate everything your associates do for the business. Nothing else can quite substitute for a few well-chosen, well-timed, sincere words of praise. They're absolutely free and worth a fortune."
>
> —Sam Walton

However, one of the most powerful, yet frequently underused, strategies to show appreciation is simply saying thank you for a job well done, especially when it is done publicly. Ideally, such recognition occurs promptly (as soon as possible after the event prompting gratitude) and spontaneously. In fact, leaders should frequently seek out opportunities to catch someone doing something right and acknowledge the behavior they wish to see more of.

Stoker (2018) agrees, noting that recognizing people for their accomplishments requires catching them doing the right things. When you observe the performance or behavior of others and say something positive, people recognize that you appreciate their efforts and value their contributions.

When showing appreciation, however, it is important to be specific. Instead of general platitudes, you could say: "I really appreciate how you dealt with that confused patient last night. You were able to de-escalate a volatile situation, sparing the patient more emotional distress and even possible harm." Or, "I know your participation on the shared governance council has brought new energy to this group and is prompting better collaboration than we have seen in some time."

Many organizations also use incentives or rewards to show appreciation. Incentive theory proposes that people are pulled toward behaviors that lead to rewards and pushed away from actions that might lead to negative outcomes (Cherry, 2019a). The use of incentives and rewards for this purpose, however, can be very challenging. While offering rewards can be motivating in some situations, researchers have found this is not always the case (Cherry, 2019b). In fact, offering excessive rewards can lead to a decrease in intrinsic motivation. Research suggests that the value of a given reward as a motivator goes down over time because employees come to expect that reward as their just due—and they quit wanting to work for it (Kazoo, n.d.). Removing the reward removes the motivated behavior. Thus, rewards typically work best in the short term. For behavior changes to last, it is usually necessary to keep the rewards coming.

In addition, some individuals erroneously believe that if a small reward results in desired behavior, a larger reward will lead to even more of the desired behavior. This simply is not true. There appears to be a perceived threshold beyond which increasing the incentive results in no additional meaning or weight. Likewise, recognizing one person's behavior and not that of another who has accomplished a similar task at a similar level promotes jealousy and can demotivate.

Working for the reward itself, rather than for the joy of the work or a sense of accomplishment, also invites corruption. For example, Wells Fargo created rewards to incentivize employees to open more checking accounts—without accountability to customers. As a result, 3.4 million accounts were opened fraudulently, creating an ongoing scandal for the company (Brumley, 2019).

"**Rewards don't bring about the changes we are hoping for, but the point here is also that something else is going on: the more rewards are used, the more they seem to be needed. ... Pretty soon, the provision of rewards becomes habitual because there seems to be no way to do without them.**"

—Alfie Kohn

Why is showing appreciation so important? Clearly, workers who feel appreciated are more engaged and have higher morale—and their productivity rises. In addition, turnover decreases. People who feel their efforts are noticed and their work makes a difference are more likely to go the extra mile in the future. So, thanking people can be good for the organization as well.

When you recognize the contributions of others, you reinforce the kind of behavior you want to see again. Employees who are typically rewarded for outstanding performance approach their jobs with greater enthusiasm and creativity. Those who do not feel appreciated often move on to other places of employment where they feel their efforts will be more appreciated.

"A person who feels appreciated will always do more than expected."

—Author unknown

"Acknowledge, Acknowledge, Acknowledge: Three valuable words in a new leader's vocabulary, and they must be said (and demonstrated) if you are going to create real leadership impact: 'I see you.'"

—Chris Westfall

"Authenticity has become the gold standard for leadership."

—Herminia Ibarra

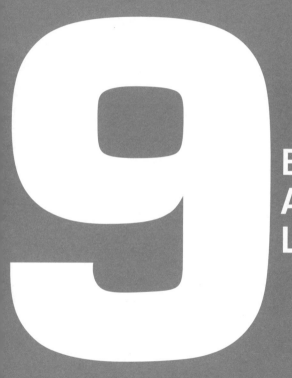

9

BE AN
AUTHENTIC
LEADER

Another strategy for creating positive work cultures is to be an authentic leader. The word *authentic* comes from the Greek word *authentikos*, which means principal or genuine (Luenendonk, 2016). Authentic leadership, then, suggests that to lead, leaders must be true to themselves and their values—and act accordingly. In other words, authentic leadership is about being true to your word and demonstrating by example so that people follow you by choice.

To be authentic, leaders must understand their purpose, practice their values, lead with their heart, establish connected relationships, and demonstrate self-discipline (Magloff, 2019). Authentic leadership is also associated with having a regard for others.

Authentic leaders are both humble and confident. For some leaders, though, finding a balance between humility and confidence can be tricky. Authentic leaders know they are worthy and fully believe in themselves and their abilities, yet they are down-to-earth, practical, and focused on implementing behaviors they can put into practice (Kruse, 2017). One of the most effective leaders I've ever met was also one of the most humble. He shared credit for his many successes and focused on empowering others to be successful. In doing so, followers felt incredibly loyal and worked hard for him and the organization to be successful.

Authentic leadership is also about predictability. Figliuolo (2018) suggests that people want to know how someone is going to react in a certain situation: A person who is predictable is more trustworthy. For example, when leaders say they are going to do something—and followers see them behave in a manner consistent with past behavior—followers are more likely to trust that those leaders will do what they say. Thus, past behavior serves as a predictor of future behavior for authentic leaders.

Authentic leadership, however, is not the same as transformational leadership, in which the leader's vision or goals are often influenced by external forces, and followers must have at least some "buy-in" of that vision. In authentic leadership, leaders' principles and conviction to act accordingly are what inspire followers.

Authentic leadership also implies a certain amount of transparency. To engender trust, authentic leaders share information with their followers whenever possible. Transparency doesn't mean, however, that "you can be held up to the light and people can see right through you" (Ibarra, 2015, para. 13). Being utterly transparent—disclosing every single thought and feeling—is both unrealistic and risky for authentic leaders.

> But [authentic leadership] does mean they are open and vulnerable about some of the challenges they may be facing or have faced in the past. They ask themselves, how can I share this challenge in a way that helps and uplifts others? They think through what they

want to say ahead of time and they share purposefully, but they're never afraid to share. (Kruse, 2017, para. 6)

Marquis and Huston (2020) caution, however, that it is naïve to believe that all leaders want to be authentic. Indeed, many are flawed, at least at times. Leaders may be deceitful or trustworthy, greedy or generous, cowardly or brave. To assume that all individuals in leadership positions are authentic is foolhardy and makes us blind to the human condition.

Lesha Reese (as cited in Forbes Coaches Council, 2018) agrees:

Leaders have long gotten away with vocally supporting policies and procedures, but their actions say otherwise. That tide will turn. With so much light being shed on unacceptable behavior in all workplaces, leaders will begin to understand they need to not only hold their teams accountable for proper behavior, but hold themselves accountable as well. (para. 7)

Sometimes, though, authentic leadership is very hard to deliver. The desire to conform and go along with others is very strong. Indeed, it takes great courage to be true to our convictions when external forces or peer pressure encourages us to do something that we feel could be inappropriate. Authentic leadership is about doing what you know to be right, even when there is a cost in doing so.

"It's no coincidence that *influence* and *influenza* come from the same root word. Real leaders are contagious. People 'catch' what they have."

–Michael Hyatt

For example, it is difficult sometimes in my current work on a hospital board to be the lone voice who speaks out against or questions something everyone else seems to support. Yet, I feel that I have earned this position on the board because of my education and the professional experiences I have gained over a lifetime and that it is my moral obligation to speak up when I question decisions. Most board members are supportive of this need to consider a different path or ask additional questions to gain more information for effective decision-making—but avoiding groupthink always involves some risk-taking and fear that others won't consider you to be a team player.

Margaret Sanger is an excellent example of an authentic nursing leader who stayed true to her values, despite high personal costs. As an early feminist and women's rights activist, Sanger coined the term "birth control" and worked toward its legalization (Biography.com editors, 2019).

In 1914, her publication *The Woman Rebel*, which promoted a woman's right to have birth control, was found to be in violation of the Comstock Act of 1873, which prohibited the trade in and circulation of "obscene and immoral materials." Rather than face a possible five-year jail sentence, Sanger fled to England but continued to work in the women's movement. She researched other forms of birth control, including diaphragms, which she later smuggled into the United States.

"A genuine leader is not a searcher for consensus but a molder of consensus."

—Martin Luther King Jr.

In 1916, Sanger opened the first birth control clinic in the United States. She was arrested during a raid of the Brooklyn clinic nine days after it opened—charged with providing information on contraception and fitting women for diaphragms. Her sentence was 30 days in jail for breaking the Comstock Act. She appealed her conviction, and although the court wouldn't overturn the earlier verdict, it made an exception in the existing law to allow doctors to prescribe contraception to their female patients for medical reasons. This was a victory for birth control and allowed Sanger to continue her work (Biography.com editors, 2019). Clearly, Sanger had conviction regarding her values, and she was willing to give up her personal liberty to see those values followed through.

Another challenge is the amount of time it takes to become an authentic leader. The process typically requires self-discovery, self-improvement, reflection, and renewal. Authentic leadership isn't about self-proclamation; it's about showing authenticity through actions and behaviors. Therefore, authentic leaders frequently question what behavior they are presenting—not by trying to be authentic but by being self-aware. This requires first achieving clarity about your inner self and then starting to showcase your actual self through your actions. Indeed, most authentic leaders need significant time and reflection to become aware of their values and priorities. They also need to develop a sense of self-worth and use their emotional intelligence to modify their approach to bring out the best in others.

"Authentic leaders have enough conviction in their values to accept that they may be misunderstood, misrepresented and maligned, yet they'll still do what's right. They've already won the toughest battle—with themselves."

—Bryan Hyde

"To be authentic, you have to know what your fears and anxieties are, and what coping mechanisms you adopted to deal with early childhood experiences that are still in effect today. You have to break through these and come to terms with yourself. You have to accept your strengths and weaknesses and be willing to share them to mentor and coach others. This is harder for some people than for others."

—Joanie Connell

Finally, authenticity may be more fluid than most people admit. The notion of adhering to one's "true self" flies in the face of much research on how people evolve with experience, discovering facets of themselves they would never have unearthed through introspection alone (Ibarra, 2015). That's why authentic leaders must be able to adapt their leadership style to changing circumstances and situations.

In the end, though, authentic leadership prowess is a cornerstone trait needed for success not just at work, but in life as well (Kruse, 2017). When leaders are emotionally self-aware, act in accordance with their stated beliefs, and build deep and loyal relationships based on trust and honesty, positive work cultures can develop and flourish.

"Good business leaders create a vision, articulate the vision, passionately own the vision, and relentlessly drive it to completion."

—Jack Welch

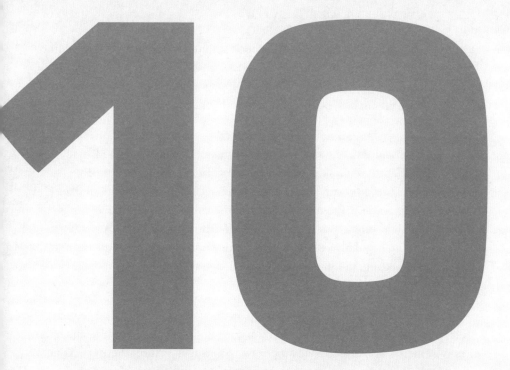

BE PASSIONATE AND PURPOSEFUL IN LOOKING TO THE FUTURE

The final strategy presented in this book for creating a positive work culture is to be passionate and purposeful in looking to the future. Looking to the future is not easy. In fact, it is quite intimidating to predict how a rapidly changing world might look different in another 5–10 years, or even longer.

Indeed, I was quite intimidated by my own first real visioning experience. In 2005, I was asked to chair a Sigma Advisory Council that was tasked with writing the preliminary draft of the strategic planning document *Vision 2020*. Working with amazing visionaries and future-oriented thinkers, however, changed my life. I emerged from the experience recognizing that vision allows us not only to better prepare for the future—it may also help us to create a preferred future. I also realized that when you cannot envision the future, you become reactive instead of proactive as a leader.

That's why vision is one of the hallmarks of leadership. Visions are about movement toward a goal, betterment, growth, or success. Thus, they communicate possibilities and solutions to both current problems and future challenges. Visions are also intentionally inclusive, painting a picture where everyone has a role that's meaningful and important (Hedges, 2018).

When leaders share strong visions, employees flock to them. These visions permeate the workplace and are manifested in the actions, beliefs, values, and goals of everyone in the organization. That's because visions are not just statements hanging on a wall; they are lived out every day at work (Heathfield, 2019).

"To lead anyone in to anything, vision is required. Without an idea of the outcome, the meandering path of a weak leader is apparent and causes apprehension and lack of confidence in one's 'followers.'"

—The Importance of Vision to Leadership

Unfortunately, many people lack vision:

> Whether unwilling or unable to imagine opportunities for change or growth, many people simply accept their current circumstances with little question or ideas for betterment. Without the drive to find a better way, forge a new path, or change the world around them in any way, most people are unwilling to put the time and effort towards being a leader. This does not mean they could not be, given the opportunity, but their complacency has already defeated them. (SocialManipulator, 2018, para. 4)

There must also, however, be an action component to that vision. Visions that are carefully developed but rarely discussed are pointless. In addition, strong visions aren't rolled out so much as woven into the fabric of the work (Hedges, 2018). Visions, then, must be brought into conversations at every opportunity.

Leadership expert Warren Bennis agrees, noting that leadership is the capacity to translate vision into reality ("Leadership," 2019). When leaders develop and share their vision, a road map is created of what needs to happen next. Kouzes and Posner (2017) note there's nothing more demoralizing than leaders who can't clearly articulate why they are doing what they are doing. That doesn't mean that leaders have all the answers. There is always some uncertainty, but success requires risk-taking, and workers need to know that their leader is anticipating the future so they won't be left behind.

"The very essence of leadership is that you have to have a vision. It's got to be a vision you articulate clearly and forcefully on every occasion."

—Theodore Hesburgh

Inspiring followers also requires *passion* because a person must have passion to have influence. Kay (2016) suggests that "leaders spread passion to others through their love of life, doing new things, taking risks, being motivated, having a sense of urgency, and reinventing self" (para. 5). Passionate people are also optimistic, have a great story, involve others, and have a simple recharge strategy. Followers look for and want to engage with people who are enthusiastic and passionate about what they are doing.

Passion, though, should never supersede *purpose*. Indeed, philosophers have long debated the tension between purpose and passion. Purpose means knowing exactly what you want to achieve and taking control of your destiny (Husary, 2019). Passion is the determination to push past all obstacles in your path to see your vision come alive. Thus, passion is about emotions, while purpose is the cause of those emotions. Or even more simply, passion is the heart, and purpose is the head (Husary, 2019). In addition, passion is typically individualistic, but purpose can be shared by all. Passion can also come and go, but purpose should be more permanent.

My guess is that we all know people who are passionate without purpose and purposeful without passion. I am drawn to passion but get discouraged when nothing is accomplished. Similarly, I am results-oriented, so I appreciate working with and for leaders who are purposeful. But when I find a leader who has both, I too can become both passionate and productive.

"You've got to follow your passion. You've got to figure out what it is you love—who you really are—And have the courage to do that. I believe that the only courage anybody ever needs is the courage to follow your own dreams."

—Oprah Winfrey

"**Purpose is the reason you journey. Passion is the fire that lights the way.**"

—Angel Chernoff

McClimon (2018) notes that if action is the result of true passion, and that passion can translate into worthwhile action, all the better. But if that direction comes from a dispassionate view that things can be better with a different approach, the resulting purpose can be a lasting noble pursuit. Thus, vision, passion, and purpose must be integrated for leaders to look to the future, anticipate needed changes, and be change champions.

When leaders look to the future, they can help organizations stay young and ever-changing. In fact, most organizations go through life stages just like people. Young organizations are all about growing and changing and thriving. Aged organizations put all their energy into maintaining the status quo; without change, they often stagnate and die.

Kodak is a great example of an aged organization. Founded in 1880 by George Eastman, Kodak became one of America's most notable companies, helping establish the market for camera film and then dominating the field. But it suffered from a variety of problems over the last four decades of its existence—almost all related to being an aged organization (Owarish, 2013).

For example, Kodak's top managers never fully grasped how the world around them was changing. They thought people would never part with hard prints, and they believed that people would never see digital photos as a direct substitute for film-based photography. So rather than accepting digital cameras in the mid-1970s as the new reality, Kodak clung to the extremely lucrative film-developing business and tried to prolong the life of film through throw-away cameras and hybrid technologies such as photo CDs (Owarish, 2013).

In essence, Kodak followed the pattern adopted by many aged organizations facing technological change. First, it tried to ignore new technology, hoping it would go away by itself. Then it openly criticized the change, suggesting it was too expensive, too slow, and too complicated. Then it tried to prolong the life of the existing technology by attempting to create synergies between the new technology and the old (like photo CDs). All these strategies delayed any serious commitment to a new order of things.

The truth is that Kodak was offered first dibs at the digital technology, but it had such an emotional attachment to its brand and its legacy that it wasted a lot of energy trying to prolong the life of existing product lines. In the end, Kodak spent an additional 15 years in "avoidance" mode until it became virtually irrelevant in the market. With only one full year of profit after 2004, Kodak filed for bankruptcy in 2012, after 131 years of being the pioneer in the film industry (Owarish, 2013).

Why is Kodak's story important to nursing leaders? It reminds us that all organizations and their leaders must continually and purposefully look to the future and embrace change if organizational cultures are to survive, much less be positive. Leaders can accomplish great things when they understand this reality, actively attempt to envision what must be done to prepare for this future, and passionately inspire others to join them on this journey.

"When you're finished changing, you're finished."

—Benjamin Franklin

REFERENCES

Advance Staff. (2018, May 29). Reducing nurse stress: Creating a culture of wellness and support. Elite Learning. Retrieved from https://www.elitecme.com/resource-center/nursing/reducing-nurse-stress-creating-a-culture-of-wellness-and-support/

Agarwal, P. (2018, August 29). How to create a positive workplace culture. *Forbes*. Retrieved from https://www.forbes.com/sites/pragyaagarwaleurope/2018/08/29/how-to-create-a-positive-work-place-culture/#4abf90244272

All Business. (2019). Boss or friend? The importance of a clearly defined working relationship. Retrieved from https://www.allbusiness.com/boss-or-friend-the-importance-of-a-clearly-defined-working-relationship-11242-1.html

The American Institute of Stress. (n.d.). Workplace stress. Retrieved from https://www.stress.org/workplace-stress/

American Nurses Association. (n.d.). Violence, incivility, & bullying. Retrieved from https://www.nursingworld.org/practice-policy/work-environment/violence-incivility-bullying/

American Nurses Association. (2017). *Executive summary. American Nurses Association health risk appraisal*. Retrieved from https://www.nursingworld.org/~4aeeeb/globalassets/practiceandpolicy/work-environment/health--safety/ana-healthriskappraisalsummary_2013-2016.pdf

Barter, A. (2017, December 7). Staying true to your core during hard times. Smart Brief. Retrieved from https://www.smartbrief.com/original/2017/12/staying-true-your-core-during-hard-times?utm_source=brief

Beard, A., McGinn, D., & Edmondson, A. (2018, November 15). Dysfunctional teams. *Harvard Business Review*. Retrieved from https://hbr.org/podcast/2018/11/dysfunctional-teams

Besner, G. (2015, July 1). Here are 4 ways to develop a culture of respect and trust. *Entrepreneur*. Retrieved from https://www.entrepreneur.com/article/247932

Biography.com Editors. (2019, April 15). Margaret Sanger biography. Biography. Retrieved from https://www.biography.com/people/margaret-sanger-9471186

Bradberry, T. (2017, January 28). 10 harsh lessons that will make you more successful. *HuffPost.* Retrieved from http://www.huffingtonpost.com/dr-travis-bradberry/10-harsh-lessons-that-wil_b_14422346.html

Branham, L., & Hirschfeld, M. (2010). *Re-engage: How America's best places to work inspire extra effort in extraordinary times.* New York, NY: McGraw-Hill Education.

Britcher, J. (2018, February 26). Replace micromanaging with macromanaging for leadership success. *Forbes.* Retrieved from https://www.forbes.com/sites/forbescoachescouncil/2018/02/26/replace-micromanaging-with-macromanaging-for-leadership-success/#5310df236f68

Brown, J. (2018, July 31). What does mutual respect look like in marriage? *Fatherly.* Retrieved from https://www.fatherly.com/love-money/marriage-advice-maintain-mutual-respect-marriage/

Brumley, J. (2019, January 14). Wells Fargo has something to prove on Tuesday morning. Retrieved from https://finance.yahoo.com/news/wells-fargo-something-prove-tuesday-180808697.html

Caldwell, B. (2018, September 9). Business kneads: The pitfalls of overworking and underperforming. Olive Group. Retrieved from https://olive.group/agency/the-pitfalls-of-overworking-and-underperforming/

Chelette, B. (2014, January 1). Why setting boundaries is so important. Retrieved from https://beatechelette.com/why-setting-boundaries-is-so-important/

Cherry, K. (2019a, May 18). The incentive theory of motivation. Verywell Mind. Retrieved from https://www.verywellmind.com/the-incentive-theory-of-motivation-2795382

Cherry, K. (2019b, May 20). What is extrinsic motivation? Verywell Mind. Retrieved from https://www.verywell.com/what-is-extrinsic-motivation-2795164

Chun, K. T. (2018, September 27). The most generous women say 'no' sometimes. *Verily.* Retrieved from https://verilymag.com/2018/09/the-importance-of-emotional-boundaries-how-to-say-no

Clark, C. (2017). *Creating and sustaining civility in nursing education* (2nd ed.). Indianapolis, IN: Sigma Theta Tau International.

Connell, J. (n.d.). Authentic leaders are great leaders—Are you? All Business. Retrieved from https://www.allbusiness.com/authentic-leaders-great-leaders-are-you-17931-1.html/2

Coolman, A. (n.d.). 3 reasons why micromanagement is a macro hindrance. B Plans. Retrieved from https://articles.bplans.com/3-reasons-why-micromanagement-is-a-macro-hindrance/

Covey, S. M. R. (2019). How the best leaders build trust. Leadership Now Project. Retrieved from https://leadershipnow.com/CoveyOnTrust.html

Craemer, M. (2018, December 21). Workplace engagement follows appreciation. *SeattlePi*. Retrieved from https://blog.seattlepi.com/workplacewrangler/2018/12/21/workplace-engagement-follows-appreciation/

Cummings, K. (2013, April 9). Trust, communication, and leadership: The three laws of influence. Association for Talent Development. Retrieved from https://www.td.org/insights/trust-communication-and-leadership-the-three-laws-of-influence

Custom Insight. (n.d.). What is employee engagement? Retrieved from http://www.custominsight.com/employee-engagement-survey/what-is-employee-engagement.asp

Daskal, D. (n.d.). How the best leaders build trust. Retrieved from https://www.lollydaskal.com/leadership/how-the-best-leaders-build-trust/

Davis, T. (2018, March 29). The workplace culture chasm: Why so many get it wrong. Knowledge@Wharton. Retrieved from http://knowledge.wharton.upenn.edu/article/building-better-work-relationships/

Douglas, A. K., & Walasik, K. J. (2018, April 12). Workplace violence prevention plans now mandatory for California hospitals and skilled nursing facilities. Epstein, Becker, Green. Retrieved from https://www.healthemploymentandlabor.com/2018/04/12/workplace-violence-prevention-plans-now-mandatory-for-california-hospitals-and-skilled-nursing-facilities/

Eades, J. (2018, December 11). Want to become a great leader in 2019? Look for these 7 signs. *Inc.* Retrieved from https://www.inc.com/john-eades/7-signs-you-are-on-your-way-to-becoming-a-great-leader-in-2019.html

Edmonds, S. C. (2018, May 24). To be the best, invest in relationships and results [Web log post]. Great Leadership. Retrieved from http://www.greatleadershipbydan.com/2018/05/to-be-best-invest-in-relationships-and.html

Figliuolo, M. (2018, April 25). Building the bonds of a high-performing team. Thought Leaders. Retrieved from http://www.thoughtleadersllc.com/2018/04/building-bonds-of-high-performing-team/

Forbes Coaches Council. (2018, January 30). 14 leadership trends that will shape organizations in 2018. *Forbes.* Retrieved from https://www.forbes.com/sites/forbescoachescouncil/2018/01/30/14-leadership-trends-that-will-shape-organizations-in-2018/#4ab51515307e

Gartenstein, D. (2019, May 10). The role of culture in leadership. Retrieved from https://bizfluent.com/info-7787192-role-culture-leadership.html

Groysberg, B., Lee, J., Price, J., & Yo-Jud Cheng, J. (2018, January/February). The leader's guide to corporate culture. *Harvard Business Review.* Retrieved from https://hbr.org/2018/01/the-culture-factor

Half, R. (2015, July 31). How to maintain professional boundaries in today's workplace. Retrieved from https://www.roberthalf.com/blog/management-tips/how-to-maintain-professional-boundaries-in-todays-workplace

Heathfield, S. M. (2018, October 29). How to demonstrate respect in the workplace. The Balance Careers. Retrieved from https://www.thebalancecareers.com/how-to-demonstrate-respect-in-the-workplace-1919376

Heathfield, S. M. (2019, March 6). Leadership vision. You can't be a real leader who people want to follow without vision. The Balance Careers. Retrieved from https://www.thebalancecareers.com/leadership-vision-1918616

Hedges, K. (2018, October 25). Don't have a leadership vision? Here's where to find it. *Forbes.* Retrieved from https://www.forbes.com/sites/work-in-progress/2018/10/25/dont-have-a-leadership-vision-heres-where-to-find-it/#554cf27a0a8a

Hockley, C. (2020). Violence in nursing: The expectations and the reality. In C. J. Huston (Ed.), *Professional issues in nursing: Challenges & opportunities* (5th ed.). Philadelphia, PA: Wolters Kluwer.

Hoff, N. (2018, May 24). Communicate clearly and openly. Smart Brief. Retrieved from https://www.smartbrief.com/original/2018/05/communicate-clearly-and-openly

Horsager, D. (2012, October 24). You can't be a great leader without trust—here's how you build it. *Forbes.* Retrieved from https://www.forbes.com/sites/forbesleadershipforum/2012/10/24/you-cant-be-a-great-leader-without-trust-heres-how-you-build-it/#13d459c4ef7a

Husary, M. (2019, January 9). Having passion and purpose. UASblog. Retrieved from https://blog.uas.aero/having-passion-and-purpose/

Huston, C. (2018, June 21). Responding to verbal abuse: Pick your battles. MedPageToday. Retrieved from https://www.medpagetoday.com/publichealthpolicy/generalprofessionalissues/73610

Hyatt, M. (2016, July 20). The 5 marks of authentic leadership. Retrieved from https://michaelhyatt.com/the-five-marks-of-authentic-leadership/

Hyde, B. (2019, January 7). Perspectives: Authentic vs. superficial leadership, can you spot the difference? *St. George News.* Retrieved from https://www.stgeorgeutah.com/news/archive/2019/01/07/perspectives-authentic-vs-superficial-leadership-can-you-spot-the-difference#.XDogbVxKiUk

Ibarra, H. (2015, January–February) The authenticity paradox. *Harvard Business Review.* Retrieved from https://hbr.org/2015/01/the-authenticity-paradox

ICA Notes. (2018, May 16). Strategies for reducing stress, anxiety, and burnout in the workplace. Retrieved from https://www.icanotes.com/2018/05/16/reducing-stress-anxiety-burnout-workplace/

Jones, C. (2018, December 21). Being buddies with the boss doesn't always pay off: Managers worry about appearing biased. *USA Today.* Retrieved from https://www.usatoday.com/story/money/2018/12/21/buddies-boss-may-cost-you-bonus-time-report-says/2280878002/

Kay, M. (2016, April 5). Top 10 leadership skills of great leaders. About Leaders. Retrieved from https://aboutleaders.com/Top-10-Leadership-Skills-of-Great-Leaders/#gs.7BNoow8B

Kazoo. (n.d.). Strategic employee rewards programs. Retrieved from https://www.kazoohr.com/strategic-employee-rewards-programs

Kluger, J. (2017, August 30). 7 signs you're dealing with a passive–aggressive person. *Time.* Retrieved from http://time.com/4916056/passive-aggressive-definition-meaning/

Kohll, A. (2018, August 14). How to build a positive company culture. *Forbes.* Retrieved from https://www.forbes.com/sites/alankohll/2018/08/14/how-to-build-a-positive-company-culture/#2dc7700249b5

Kohn, A. (2016, February 17). Quotes from: "Punished by rewards: The trouble with gold stars, incentive plans, A's, praise, and other bribes" by Alfie Kohn. Key Steps to Success Consulting. Retrieved from https://www.keystepstosuccess.com/2016/02/quotes-from-punished-by-rewards-the-trouble-with-gold-stars-incentive-plans-as-praise-and-other-bribes-by-alfie-cohn/

Kouzes, J. M., & Posner, B. Z. (2017). *The leadership challenge: How to make extraordinary things happen in organizations* (6th ed.). Hoboken, NJ: Wiley.

Kruse, K. (2017, June 20). 5 keys to authentic leadership. *Forbes.* Retrieved from https://www.forbes.com/sites/kevinkruse/2017/06/20/5-keys-to-authentic-leadership/#38fc210b14da

Lampert, L. (2016, March 1). Depression in nurses: The unspoken epidemic. *Minority Nurse.* Retrieved from https://minoritynurse.com/depression-in-nurses-the-unspoken-epidemic/

Lancer, D. (2016). What are personal boundaries? How do I get some? Psych Central. Retrieved from https://psychcentral.com/lib/what-are-personal-boundaries-how-do-i-get-some/

Lauby, S. (2019, January 4). Give employees recognition and rewards that matter—Friday distraction. HR Bartender. Retrieved from https://www.hrbartender.com/2019/employee-engagement/recognition-rewards/

Leadership. (2019). *Psychology Today.* Retrieved from https://www.psychologytoday.com/us/basics/leadership

Lipman, V. (2019, January 9). Workplace trend: Stress is on the rise. *Forbes.* Retrieved from https://www.forbes.com/sites/victorlipman/2019/01/09/workplace-trend-stress-is-on-the-rise/#175933366e1b

Llopis, G. (2013, November 4). The 4 most effective ways leaders solve problems. *Forbes.* Retrieved from https://www.forbes.com/sites/glennllopis/2013/11/04/the-4-most-effective-ways-leaders-solve-problems/#3f9be3d44f97

Locke, L., Bromley, G., & Federspiel, K. A. (2018, May). Patient violence: It's not all in a day's work. *American Nurse Today, 13*(5). Retrieved from https://www.americannursetoday.com/patient-violence/

Luenendonk, M. (2016, August 18). Authentic leadership guide: Definitions, qualities, pros & cons, examples. Cleverism. Retrieved from https://www.cleverism.com/authentic-leadership-guide/

Magloff, L. (2019). What is an authentic leadership style? *Houston Chronicle*. Retrieved from https://smallbusiness.chron.com/authentic-leadership-style-10866.html

Magnuson, D. (2017, July 5). The abuse of micromanagement in the workplace & job performance. Career Trend. Retrieved from https://careertrend.com/about-6670994-abuse-micromanagement-workplace-job-performance.html

Mann, C. (2018, January 1). Violence against nurses. *Kansas Nurse, 93*(1), 14–17.

Marlin, D. (2017, April 21). 27 quotes to change how you think about problems. *Entrepreneur*. Retrieved from https://www.entrepreneur.com/article/288957

Marquis, B., & Huston, C. (2020). *Leadership roles and management functions in nursing* (10th ed). Philadelphia, PA: Wolters Kluwer.

Martin, S. (2018a, June 20). How to set boundaries with an alcoholic or addict. Psych Central. Retrieved from https://blogs.psychcentral.com/imperfect/2017/08/how-to-set-boundaries-with-an-alcoholic-or-addict/

Martin, S. (2018b, January 7). What are healthy boundaries and why do I need them? Psych Central. Retrieved from https://blogs.psychcentral.com/imperfect/2016/05/what-are-healthy-boundaries-why-do-i-need-boundaries/

Mason Jubb, J., & Baack, C. J. (2019, January). Verbal de-escalation for clinical practice safety. *American Nurse Today, 14*(1). Retrieved from https://www.americannursetoday.com/verbal-de-escalation-safety/

McFarlin, K. (n.d.). How to address issues & problems in the workplace. *Houston Chronicle*. Retrieved from https://smallbusiness.chron.com/address-issues-problems-workplace-10186.html

McClimon, T. J. (2018, November 12). Purpose vs. passion in leadership: Which do you need most? *Forbes*. Retrieved from https://www.forbes.com/sites/timothyjmcclimon/2018/11/12/purpose-vs-passion-in-leadership-which-do-you-need-most/#14432f2236b4

Meyer, P. (2019, February 15). Apple Inc.'s organizational culture & its characteristics (an analysis). Panmore Institute. Retrieved from http://panmore.com/apple-inc-organizational-culture-features-implications

Mind Tools. (n.d.). Building trust inside your team. Ways to improve team cohesion. Retrieved from https://www.mindtools.com/pages/article/building-trust-team.htm

Molloy, A. (2017, July 21). Why people who are micromanaged eventually quit. Collective Hub. Retrieved from https://collectivehub.com/2017/07/why-people-who-are-micromanaged-eventually-quit/

Mulholland, B. (2018, July 20). Don't micromanage: How it destroys your team and how to avoid it. Process Street. Retrieved from https://www.process.st/micromanage/

Naseer, T. (n.d.). How leaders are creating engagement in today's workplaces. Tanveer Naseer Leadership. Retrieved from https://www.tanveernaseer.com/what-fortune-500-leaders-are-doing-to-create-employee-engagement/

Owarish, F. (2013). Strategic leadership of technology: Lessons learned. E-Leader Singapore. Retrieved from https://www.g-casa.com/conferences/singapore12/papers/Owarish-2.pdf

Pearson, C. (2013, November 22). 10 steps to halt the contagion of workplace incivility. Thunderbird School of Global Management. Retrieved from https://thunderbird.asu.edu/knowledge-network/workplace-incivility

Pettit, J. (2018, December 4). Leadership tips for 2019! CU Insight. Retrieved from https://www.cuinsight.com/leadership-tips-for-2019.html

Reilly, F. (2017, February 14). Maintaining healthy boundaries when being of service. The Event Chronicle. Retrieved from http://www.theeventchronicle.com/media/informational/maintaining-healthy-boundaries-service/

Reuter, G. (2018, December 18). Is micromanaging an effective management model? LBi Software. Retrieved from http://www.lbisoftware.com/blog/micromanaging-as-management-model/

Reynolds, J. (2017, January 25). 15 team-building activities to build trust among coworkers. TINYpulse. Retrieved from https://www.tinypulse.com/blog/team-building-activity-trust

Rogers, K. (2018, July–August). Do your employees feel respected? *Harvard Business Review*. Retrieved from https://hbr.org/2018/07/do-your-employees-feel-respected

Ryan, L. (2016, October 19). Ten unmistakable signs of a toxic culture. *Forbes*. Retrieved from https://www.forbes.com/sites/lizryan/2016/10/19/ten-unmistakable-signs-of-a-toxic-culture/#637615a0115f

Scott, S. (2019). Team building activities focusing on communication. *Houston Chronicle*. Retrieved from https://smallbusiness.chron.com/team-building-activities-focusing-communication-10561.html

SocialManipulator. (2018, November 19). The importance of vision to leadership [Web log post]. Retrieved from https://strategicmanipulation.wordpress.com/2018/11/19/the-importance-of-vision-to-leadership/

Society for Human Resource Management. (2017, April 24). 2017 employee job satisfaction and engagement: The doors of opportunity are open. Retrieved from https://www.shrm.org/hr-today/trends-and-forecasting/research-and-surveys/pages/2017-job-satisfaction-and-engagement-doors-of-opportunity-are-open.aspx

Solomon, M. (2018, October 5). Does culture really eat strategy for lunch? How leadership and company culture interact. *Forbes*. Retrieved from https://www.forbes.com/sites/micahsolomon/2018/10/05/does-culture-really-eat-strategy-for-lunch-how-leadership-and-company-culture-interact/#1fde31903f0d

Spath, T., & Dahnke, C. (n.d.) What is civility? The Institute for Civility in Government. Retrieved from https://www.instituteforcivility.org/who-we-are/what-is-civility/

Stoker, J. R. (2018, July 17). Tips for supercharging your leadership credibility. Smart Brief. Retrieved from https://www.smartbrief.com/original/2018/07/tips-supercharging-your-leadership-credibility

Tartakovsky, M. (2018). 10 ways to build and preserve better boundaries. Psych Central. Retrieved from https://psychcentral.com/lib/10-way-to-build-and-preserve-better-boundaries/

Thompson, R. (2019, January). What if you're the bully? *American Nurse Today*, *14*(1). Retrieved from https://www.americannursetoday.com/what-if-youre-the-bully/

Wallen, J. (2015, January 5). 6 big dangers of micromanagement. Pluralsight. Retrieved from https://www.pluralsight.com/blog/business-professional/why-micromanagement-is-bad

Westfall, C. (2019, January 8). 10 team-building tips for new leaders. *Forbes.* Retrieved from https://www.forbes.com/sites/chriswestfall/2019/01/08/ten-team-building-tips-new-leaders/#c6e434f52337

Wojciechowski, M. (2018, April 5). Emotional rescue: How to protect yourself from stressful work experiences. *Minority Nurse.* Retrieved from https://minoritynurse.com/emotional-rescue-how-to-protect-yourself-from-stressful-work-experiences/

Work Points Play. (2019). The five trends that will impact employee recognition in 2019. Retrieved from https://workpointsplay.com/blog/2019-employee-recognition-trends

Workplace Bullying Institute. (2019). The WIB definition of workplace bullying. Retrieved from http://www.workplacebullying.org/individuals/problem/definition/

Yazdi, M. (2019, January 2). 8 tips to help bring the magic back to nursing in 2019. Nurse.org. Retrieved from https://nurse.org/articles/tips-to-overcome-nurse-burnout-2019/

INDEX

A

American Nurses Association, 22, 27
Apple Inc., 8
appreciation
  effective forms of, 91–94
  importance of, 90–97
  rewards and, 93–95
  timing of recognition, 93
  values and, 91
  words of praise, 92–93
authentic leadership
  difficulties in achieving, 102, 104
  fluidity of, 109
  Margaret Sanger as example of, 104, 106
  predictability of, 101
  qualities of authentic leaders, 100–109
  as time-intensive process, 106
  vs. transformational leadership, 101
  transparency and, 101–102

B

bias, perceptions of, 38–39
boundaries
  characteristics of, 30
  confusion about, 30
  emotional boundaries, 33, 35
  feedback and, 31
  personal *vs.* professional relationships, 36, 38–39
  physical boundaries, 31
  self-care, 36
  in sharing with coworkers, 33
  social media, 30, 33, 34
  work/life balance, 35–36
bullying
  definitions of, 21–22
  impact of, 26

C

civility
  characteristics of, 21

W–Z